Fructose Malabsorption
The Survival Guide

Debra & Bob Ledford

ISBN: 978-0-9840777-0-0

To order additional books, please contact:

www.fructosemalabsorptionhelp.com
or
Ledford Publishing
P.O. Box 6756
Brookings, OR 97415

Send comments, questions, or information to:
help@fructosemalabsorptionhelp.com

Debra's Dedication

To my husband and co-author, Bob, without whose love and support, this book, and my current state of wellness, would not have been possible.

To my mom, Deretha Rard, who has always supported me in my endeavors.

And to my dad, Paul Rard, I hope you are proud of our accomplishment. I miss you.

Bob's Dedication

To my wife, Debra, for her willingness to open her mind, and her eagerness to share what she has learned in order to help others.

Special Thanks to:
Jill Cairns-Gallimore,
Suzie Biggs, and Judy May-Lopez for their editing assistance.

Table of Contents

5

Introduction

When I was first diagnosed with Fructose Malabsorption (FM), the extreme frustration we felt trying to find sources of information was exasperating. Numerous hours on the internet produced insignificant help, only confusing us more. The few lists available were conflicting, without explanations. We quickly saw the need for a single, reliable source.

After many, perhaps thousands of hours of research, we have compiled what we feel is the most comprehensive resource to date for the FM sufferer. In this book we have attempted to address: questions asked by the FMer, lists, resources, dealing with the effects, recipes, our viewpoints, and much more.

If you have comments, questions, corrections, recommendations, or other helpful information, please e-mail us at help@fructosemalabsorptionhelp.com. We may include helpful information in future editions of this book.

Disclaimer

This is a book written by an FM family as support for FMer's and their families. We are not medical personnel and are not qualified to dispense advice, medical or otherwise. The information contained herein is a compilation of research and our opinions, not meant to be taken as medical advice. We urge you to consult your physician and get tested before implementation of anything contained in this book.

My Story – Part One

As a preface to my story I would like to advise my readers that out of necessity of subject matter I will be sharing very personal information. I do this, not from lack of sensitivity or discretion, but to better facilitate understanding of this condition and its resulting effect on me.

Approximately two and a half years ago, I began my journey of discovery into the cause behind the stomach problems I was experiencing. What had previously been chronically irritating problems had become acutely disruptive problems. Stomach pain had become almost constant, antacids were purchased in large quantities, uncontrollable flatulence (passing gas) was a source of humiliation, and severe constipation was making me ill.

The constipation seemed to be the primary source of my misery; therefore I began by focusing on it. With avoidance of laxatives being advisable due to the physical dependence which is easily developed by regular use, I began with more natural and pleasant methods. I love fruit, so I focused on oranges, which had previously been the only fruit which had ever actually aided me with this problem. Adding prune juice, despite the fact that it had never given me the same results digestively which it apparently does the general population, helped to appease those who were trying to advise me. I also focused on roughage, or high-fiber foods, grains and vegetables which are known to aid digestion. Of course I increased my water intake, although I tend to drink large amounts normally. Additionally, I avoided meats, cheese, milk, and other products which might be slowing my processing facilities. Despite all of this, matters just got worse.

As a lifelong opponent of "fad" diets, desperate describes what I was feeling and my next course of action. I resorted to a liquid-only diet in an attempt to "cleanse." Obviously, in addition to broth and plenty of water, this meant mostly fruit and vegetable juices. As a health-conscious parent, I had always required all juice consumed in our home to be 100% juice, without added sweeteners or flavors so be assured, this juice was actually juice. All to no avail, the earth still moved, but I did not.

For those who have never known the experience of chronic and severe constipation, after about three weeks of "nothing," the toxins accumulate within the body to the extent one actually becomes quite ill, take-to-your-bed type ill. I was nearing this. Extreme situations...as they say, so I bought what I felt would be the strongest over-the-counter laxative I could get, Extra-Strength Ex-Lax. I took the maximum dosage for a full week. Not only was I surprised by the fact that I did not get the usual cramping such products cause, but this also resulted in an insignificant amount of action.

After making an appointment with my internist and having blood tests, his nurse telephoned, stating the tests were all normal and the doctor had called in a prescription, for a laxative...I would not need to return. I said "No, thank you." I was not interested in treating only the symptoms; I wanted to know the cause. I then asked for a referral to a gastroenterologist, a specialist of the digestive tract. A few days later I went for my appointment.

At the gastroenterologist's, the nurse practitioner took an extensive medical history, as well as the details of my current problem. More tests were ordered to discover if the acid reflux had caused esophageal damage and to rule out such things as crohns disease and colitis, both hereditary diseases which my brother was diagnosed with at the age of twenty-one. However, she felt there was a good possibility I might have fructose malabsorption. After being told it is an "intolerance" to fructose, I was determined this was not my problem, after all, I love fruits and vegetables.

After a wonderfully liberating week of a combination of different laxatives, I went back for more tests, one of which tested for fructose malabsorption. The good news that all the tests showed me to be perfectly healthy was overshadowed by the fact that the nurse practitioner had been correct, I have fructose malabsorption.

What is Fructose Malabsorption?

With fructose malabsorption (FM), erroneously known as fructose intolerance or dietary fructose intolerance, fructose, a naturally occurring sugar found in fruit, vegetables, and honey, is not absorbed by the small intestine. Normally, fructose is absorbed by the small intestine using enterocytes - intestinal absorptive cells - to break up molecules and transport them into the tissues. In those for whom this protein is either missing or inactive, the fructose continues to the large intestine, where it is fermented by intestinal bacteria becoming short chain fatty acids and the gases carbon dioxide, methane, and hydrogen.

You may be wondering why you have never heard of FM before. It is a fairly recent diagnosis. This does not mean it is the latest popular diagnosis. This means until recently, it was unknown what caused this group of symptoms.

This is important...*fructose malabsorption should not be confused with hereditary fructose* *intolerance* (HFI), a rare, life-threatening disorder in which fructose is absorbed within the small intestine but is not metabolized by the liver. This is a completely different condition unrelated to FM. People with this disorder require a completely fructose-free diet.

Diagnosis

A diagnosis of FM is done by a simple breath hydrogen test. After fasting for eight to twelve hours the patient begins the test by blowing into a small bag, which is then sealed, for a baseline sample, followed by drinking a solution of fructose water. The patient will then continue the process of blowing into a new small bag every twenty minutes for a period of time from two to five hours. I did this for three hours. After completion of the test, the bags are sent to the lab for analysis. This test can also be done using a machine which will give immediate results, though few doctors have it available, while the "bag" version is quite inexpensive and readily available for any doctor's office to administer. The patient is considered to have FM if the hydrogen levels in the samples are twenty points or more above the baseline sample level in two or more of the samples. My highest reading was 116. This test is simple and non-invasive, with its only negatives being the amount of time involved and the reaction to the fructose for those with FM.

Sample	Time	Clock	ppm H2
Baseline	0	8:35	0
1	20 minutes	8:55	0
2	40 minutes	9:15	29
3	1 hour	9:35	116
4	80 minutes	9:55	47
5	100 minutes	10:15	38
6	2 hours	10:35	36
7	140 minutes	10:55	57
8	160 minutes	11:15	29
9	3 hours	11:35	9

Copy of my Breath Hydrogen Test Results

Caution: Anyone suspected of having Hereditary Fructose Intolerance (HFI) should not have a fructose breath hydrogen test before undergoing tests for HFI since this could result in a serious hypoglycemic reaction.

As a result of the nutritional and dietary challenges faced by an FMer, I am completely baffled as to why anyone would self-diagnose this condition and not have a breath hydrogen test done. Aside from the many serious conditions which may go undetected with an improper "opinion" of FM, this is not easy to live with. Get tested!

Remember, you are in charge of your body. If you suspect you have FM and your physician is resistant to testing, you are allowed to be insistent. Where would I be if I had accepted the initial prescribed laxatives and not insisted on a referral to a gastroenterologist? The diet for FM is too restrictive and to difficult to live with to accept an "opinion" of FM without testing. So be insistent!

One of the difficulties in diagnosing FM without a breath hydrogen test is the vast array of seemingly unrelated symptoms. Additional complications arise when one considers that different foods trigger different symptoms. While one food may produce the classic stomach cramps, another initiates puffiness. Though I am reluctant to repeat myself, I will...get tested!

Symptoms of Fructose Malabsorption

Symptoms of FM include:

(Not all FMer's experience all symptoms.)

- Stomach pain
- Flatulence (passing gas)
- Acid indigestion/heartburn/acid reflux
- Diarrhea / constipation
- Bloating – this occurs internally as well as externally, making breathing labored and blocking sinuses
- Burping
- Bad Breath

Also associated with FM:

- Headaches
- "Fuzzy" head
- Fatigue
- Depression / mood disorders
- Sugar cravings
- Inability to lose / gain weight
- Hemorrhoids

- Concentration difficulties
- Dark circles under eyes
- Lack of sense of smell
- Difficulty sleeping

Studies have also shown the following to be associated with FM:

- Iron deficiency
- High triglycerides
- Folic acid deficiency
- Elevated LDL cholesterol
- Zinc deficiency

With the exception of iron (which for me is on the low end of normal) and folic acid, (of which I am unaware), every item listed here describes me. Learning of this condition and researching it has provided answers to many questions. The "treatment" has brought both relief and a compounding of problems.

Treatment for Fructose Malabsorption

The good news: There are no medications to take, surgery involved, or repeated visits to the doctor. The bad news: FM is treated solely by dietary restrictions which are very unclear and individualized. Unlike individuals who are lactose intolerant, FMers do not have the option of taking an enzyme to alleviate their condition. Fructose is a mono-saccharide, so it cannot be broken down further by taking an enzyme or any other medication. It is already at its basic form. Lactose is a disaccharide, allowing those who are intolerant to take an enzyme to further break it down to a mono-saccharide, thus rendering it absorbable.

Researching FM on the internet will offer a limited amount of information which is very conflicting. Books on the subject seem almost non-existent. So few people are familiar with FM that it is difficult to find a dictician or nutritionist qualified to help.

Take care when searching for a dietician or nutritionist to "interview" them before making an appointment. Ask how many clients they have worked with who have FM. I spent $70 dollars for a consultation with a nutritionist-only to discover she knew less than I did. When I made the appointment, I had asked if she was familiar with FM and had been told "Yes." During our consultation she used the same printouts I had gotten from researching FM on the internet when first diagnosed. She appeared not to know the difference between FM and HFI. After asking how many clients she had with FM, I discovered I was the first. It seems her familiarity came from her conversation with the person who had referred me to her!

I was told by the gastroenterologist's nurse practitioner to begin with at least two weeks of totally fructose-free diet, and was given a small amount of information on the diet for HFI, which was a copy of what I had already found on the internet. This diet is very difficult. It does not allow any fructose or sugar. Reading labels will prove this comes close to restricting a diet to unprocessed meats, dairy, and fresh produce…most of which cannot be eaten.

I stayed on this diet for about six weeks hoping the extra time would allow my body to "heal" from some of what I had been through. Then I slowly began adding items to see what I could tolerate or was no problem.

A surprising advantage of this restriction came in the form of a relatively flat tummy. I had been wondering why I had gained so much in the entire stomach area, especially just below my bra. I had a "shelf" which distended out about two inches. Not only did my "shelf" go away, but so did the bulge on down my torso. I felt skinny! It was as though I had lost 10 pounds. This result only took about a week. It was not weight, it was bloat. I just needed to clean my system. Now it is quite simple to see if I am reacting to something, I have a shelf.

Before going any further, let me give you my definitions of terms I use to differentiate between foods.

- Can eat – foods which cause no adverse reaction.

- Tolerate – foods for which I show no immediate reaction, but will wake up the next morning (if it was dinner) with symptoms. This is usually accompanied by swelling, lethargy, etc. Obviously, I don't tolerate them well.

- Can not eat – foods which, within ten to twenty minutes after consumption, will cause acid indigestion, pain, gas, or in people who have diarrhea problems, a dash to the restroom. These symptoms will then be followed the next day by other symptoms such as bloating and headache and may last up to three days, though it may take as long as a week to feel "normal" again. Some report it takes even longer to achieve normalcy.

The wonderful thing about living with FM is…after eating right for a short time, the length of which seems to differ for each FMer (usually three days to two weeks), the symptoms disappear. No waking in the middle of the night suffering with gas pains, no constipation/diarrhea, no fuzzy head, no high triglycerides….well, you get the idea. This is an amazing detail for a person who has lived with multiple, seemingly unrelated, symptoms. Not only does it feel wonderful physically, but the vast mental and emotional relief involved is extremely reassuring. Despite what some had speculated, I'm really *not* a hypochondriac!

The Diet

Due to the nature of food intolerances, different people have different levels of tolerance to offensive foods. While some cannot tolerate any, others react only to large quantities. This makes a defined diet even more difficult. Ask ten different FMer's and you will receive ten different lists of foods. Compound this by the conflicting information available and life for the FMer can be quite frustrating.

If you are also lactose intolerant, I feel for you. Finding appropriate foods will be even more difficult. If you are a vegetarian, you may decide, as many have, out of sheer necessity to add at least some meat to your diet. I would be interested to hear how those of you who fit into these categories have faired.

Most foods contain a mixture of fructose and glucose. According to research[1], it is the ratio of this mixture, restricted to fructose never higher than glucose, with which the FMer needs to be concerned.

"Absorption is enhanced by co-ingestion with glucose, since glucose uptake stimulates additional transport pathways for fructose absorption in the small intestinal epithelial cell"[1]. As a result "people with fructose malabsorption need to avoid foods high in free fructose, but can manage those with balanced concentrations of fructose and glucose (or a greater concentration of glucose)"[1]. As a way of proving this "19 patients with an abnormal breath test and symptoms following fructose were reexamined after a load with equimolar concentrations of glucose and fructose. Hydrogen breath test was normal in all of them, none developed abdominal discomfort."[3] This fructose-glucose ratio component reveals that FMer's can eat fruit, but only in limited quantities. "In addition to excess fructose foods, those high in the balanced sugars may also be problematic when consumed in large amounts as these provide a high fructose load. For example, an orange is in equal balance of fructose and glucose so is safe to eat, however, orange juice is concentrated, with one glass containing up to six oranges, so this should be limited to only one-third glass in one sitting (equivalent to the juice from one serving of fruit)"[1].   In other words, be sure the balance of fructose to glucose is higher in glucose, and then be sure to limit the quantity.

When I first discovered this, it had been a year since I had consumed any fruit. Okay, I had eaten one grape and it doubled me over within ten minutes of eating it. Anyway, the ratio idea made perfect sense to me since citrus fruits have been the only fruit I had ever eaten which helped to loosen my digestive system.

After learning I might be able to eat an orange I tried a half of a small one. That first bite was amazing! It was as though I had bitten into a juicy, flavorful piece of heaven. I closed my eyes and savored every nuance of it: from the glorious aroma, to the beady texture, to the luscious juiciness, to the explosive flavor. Eating that orange was a definite pinnacle of dining experiences. *Chocolate* has never tasted that good. Even better, there was no reaction!

An exception to the fructose-glucose ratio is found in foods containing polyols, of which sorbitol is the most common. Maltitol and isomalt are also types of polyols. "Their absorption is not accelerated by co-ingestion with glucose but seems to be worse when given concomitantly with glucose"[1]. Sorbitol is an alternative sweetener commonly used in diabetic foods. Polyols are also added to chewing gum to prevent tooth decay because they are not broken down by the bacteria in the mouth as is sugar. Unfortunately, it is also found in "stone" fruits, such as plums, apricots, and cherries. Consequently, despite the favorable ratio of these fruits, they are not appropriate for those with FM.

The glucose/fructose ratio presents another conflict. Some foods which are clearly unacceptable for me, should theoretically be acceptable by their ratio. Of course, this is complemented by foods which are acceptable for me, but should not be, according to their ratio. Once again, there is no magic formula; trial and error is the best way to form your own personal list. The fructose/glucose ratio is a good place to start though.

Wheat is another problem with FM. "A person can suffer from wheat intolerance but not fructose malabsorption. However, if they have fructose malabsorption, they will have problems with high intakes of wheat" [6]. However, "Wheat is a problem in large amounts, i.e. when it is the main ingredient in a product"[1]. Hence, bread, pasta, and pastries *may* be problematic for those with FM. Herein lies some of the conflict; many sources list pasta as a "safe" food. The key phrases here are "high intakes" and "main ingredient."

Why is wheat not safe? Wheat is in the fructan category. Technically, these are chains of fructose molecules ending with a glucose molecule. In English, they allow the plant to thrive in low temperatures and during drought. Though tolerance for these vary, they are not usually acceptable for FMer's. Wheat, spelt, brown rice (the hull of the rice), onions and their family, are a few of the fructans to avoid. See the "Fructan Foods" list, page 167.

I have discovered that it is best for me to stay away from the whole-wheat variety of pastas and breads. If wheat pasta is problematic, the easiest way to get around it is by using rice pasta. Limiting the quantity I eat also helps. Rather than having a whole sandwich I limit myself to one-half a sandwich. This also helps me to eat less at one time.

Quantity restriction is important for those with FM. In addition to eating limited amounts of those permissible foods with a "glucose higher than fructose" ratio, quantity in general should be limited. In the digestive tract "the contents comprise solid, liquid and gas components and dietary factors can influence all of these".[1] The conclusion may then be drawn that, since it is difficult for the FM sufferer to avoid problematic foods entirely and there is limited capacity within the digestive tract, larger quantities of food coupled with liquid and gas will be more likely to result in pain.

I have found the above to be quite accurate. So much so that I have been trying to restrict myself to six "mini-meals" rather than any large meals, regardless of what I eat. Thankfully, this seems to be helping. As an added advantage to this, the "experts" say it is generally supposed to be a healthier way to eat.

Sugars & Sweeteners

There are many different types of sugar, each from different sources, with different possible consequences for the FMer.

I believe the reason my FM problem became so acute, necessitating diagnosis, is that when we ran out of table sugar at work I discovered Splenda ® and began using it instead of sugar. Splenda ® and FM do not get along.

As with most foods, each FMer must determine which sugars they can tolerate and to what extent. For instance, I enjoy organic cane sugar, which has a 50:50 ratio of fructose/glucose, but as with all sugars, quantities must be limited. It is my understanding many FMer's cannot tolerate even small quantities of table sugar. As the table below will reveal, this may be due to eating table sugar made with beet sugar rather than cane sugar.

I frequently have people ask me if I have to follow a diabetic diet. The answer is…absolutely not.

Diabetics must restrict their intake of glucose, thus a frequent substitute for sugar in their diets is sorbitol. Conversely, the FMer must avoid sorbitol completely and requires an appropriate fructose/glucose ratio (with glucose being higher). Hence, our diets are not even closely related. If you are a diabetic and an FMer, you will definitely need to work with your dietician.

Be careful about foods which are "sugar free," they frequently contain artificial sweeteners. Also be cautious with foods labeled "fat free" or "low fat," which frequently add sugar or artificial sweetener to compensate for the loss of fat. As always, read the labels.

The following chart is an adaptation of the "Sugars & Sweeteners" chart on the Boston University website for hereditary fructose intolerance (HFI) [11]. (Used by permission) The original chart includes a wide variety of sugars and sweeteners which are not common and for those of us hoping to simplify and understand, can be rather overwhelming so we have provided this condensed version listing the more common sweeteners. Additionally, since the original chart was designed for HFI patients (thus resulting in more confusion for the FMer), we have revised it somewhat for the FMer. The tolerance column has been changed to reflect the FMer's tolerance as gleaned from my experience coupled with comments from other FMer's on the internet. Remember, tolerance levels may differ and quantity is a factor. Determine your own tolerance levels. The "**?**" in the tolerance column is an indication that tolerance seems to vary widely.

Sugar Sweetener	Description	Tolerance
Agave Syrup	From the blue agave cactus. Commonly used in Tex-Mex foods, tequila, margaritas, soft drinks. High in fructose.	No
Aspartame	Sugar substitute known as Equal, NutraSweet, NutraTase. FDA approved. Scientifically studied in depth. Some may be sensitive to headaches. Derived from amino acids.	No
Barley Malt Syrup	From sprouted grains of barley, kiln dried and cooked with water.	?
Beet Sugar	Sucrose. Same structure as cane sugar, but may produce different product results because of .05 differences in minerals and proteins. More common in Europe than the U.S	No

Brown Rice Syrup	Made from brown rice. High protein content. Likely contains sucrose.	?
Brown Sugar	Sucrose coated with molasses.	No
Cane Sugar	Sucrose. Table sugar.	Yes
Corn Starch	Derived from corn. Composed of straight or branched chains of glucose.	No
Corn Sugar	Produced from corn starch. Contains glucose and maltose molecules.	No
Corn Syrup	Glucose and water. Usually produced from cornstarch. The problem is that in making the syrup, it may have either maltose and/or fructose added.	No
Corn Syrup Solids	Dried glucose syrup.	No

Confectioners Sugar	Sucrose. A chemical combination of glucose and fructose.	Yes
Date Sugar	Made from dried, pulverized dates. Likely contains sucrose.	No
Dextrin	Glucose molecules linked together in chains. Does not break down to pure dextrose.	Yes
Dextrose	Single glucose molecule. Simple sugar.	Yes
Evaporated Cane Sugar	Sucrose. Another name for sugar cane juice.	Yes
Fructose	Simple sugar of fructose molecules. Sometimes called fruit sugar. Made of 6 carbons.	No
Fruit Juice Sweeteners	Derived from grapes, apples or pears, heated to reduce water leaving a sweeter more concentrated juice. Almost pure fructose.	No

Glucose	Simple sugar. The chemical sugar structure of blood sugar. Made of 6 carbons.	Yes
Granulated sugar	Table sugar. Sucrose. Can be tolerated only if it is pure cane sugar, not beet sugar.	?
High Fructose Corn Syrup (HFCS)	Enzymetically converted from corn syrup to contain 42% - 90% fructose. Raises triglyceride levels and may increase risk of heart disease. See the chapter on HFCS.	No
Honey	Natural syrup containing about 35% glucose, 40% fructose, 25 % water	No
Inverted Sugar	Created by combining sugar syrup with cream of tarter or lemon juice and heating, breaking sucrose down to components glucose and fructose.	No
Isoglucose	Another name for High Fructose Corn Syrup (HFCS).	No
Isomalt	Polyol	No

Levulose	Contains fructose.	No
Maltitol	Sugar alcohol form of maltose (glucose). This is a polyol.	No
Maltose	Linked glucose molecules that rapidly break down to glucose in the intestine.	Yes
Maple Syrup	Mostly sucrose. Contains some invert sugar.	No
Molasses	By-product of sugar cane with 24% water. Fructose level varies. Three kinds. Light (sweetest), Medium (darker and less sweet), Blackstrap (very dark, slightly sweet with distinctive flavor. Good source of calcium and iron)	No
Molasses Sugar	Dark muscovado sugar with extra molasses.	No
Raffinose	A trisaccharide found in grains, legumes and some vegetables. Gas forming.	?

Raw Sugar	Sucrose. Equal parts glucose and fructose, a chemical combination of glucose and fructose.	Yes
Saccharin	Sugar substitute. Not as commonly used as in the past. Known as Sweet N' Low, Sugar Twin, Sucryl, Featherweight. FDA approved. More than 6 servings per day may increase bladder cancer risk. (No longer approved for use in Canada)	No
Sorbitol	Sugar alcohol. Common in fruits, particularly skin of ripe berries, cherries and plums. Used in sugar free foods. Causes diarrhea. Converted back to fructose. This is a polyol.	No
Splenda	A sugar substitute. This is a chemically modified sucrose molecule that □china be digested.	No
Stevia	Natural sweetener from a South American plant. 30 % sweeter than sugar. Used extensively in Japan, China, Korea, Israel, Brazil and Paraguay with no side effects reported. Known as Stevioside. Has not been rigorously tested for safety. No consistent manufacturing regulations.	Yes
Sucralose	Chemical name for Splenda, a sugar substitute. Large molecule not digested.	No

Sucrose	Naturally occurring sugar made from sugar cane or sugar beets. Commonly referred to as sugar and table sugar. Chemical combination of glucose and fructose. Tolerated if from cane but not from beets.	?
Sucrose Syrups	Also known as Refiner's syrup. By product of sugar refining. 18% water, 1 part sucrose to two parts invert sugar.	No
Sugar	Common name for sucrose, a chemical combination of glucose and fructose.	Yes
Xylitol	Sugar alcohol. Obtained from fruits and berries. Also from birch trees and known as birch sugar. May causes diarrhea.	?

High Fructose Corn Syrup

Read a few labels next time you go to the grocery store. There is a very good chance you will see high fructose corn syrup (HFCS) on most of them. It is in the soda you drink, many canned fruits, cereal, yogurt, bread, peanut butter, and the list goes on and on. Technically, it is "enzyme-catalyzed isomerization of glucose (dextrose) to the sweeter sugar, fructose (levulose)"[2]. This, stated in somewhat slightly more comprehensible English, "undergone enzymatic processing in order to increase their fructose content and are then mixed with pure corn syrup (100% glucose)"[4] Unfortunately (in my opinion), "Subsequent development of separation processes for enriching the fructose content not only allowed production of syrups with higher fructose content than could be produced by enzymatic action alone, but ultimately allowed the manufacture of pure crystalline fructose from starch."[2] HFCS was developed in 1957, refined in the 1970s, and began a rapid introduction to foods from 1975 to 1985 (see chart at the end of this chapter).

One source actually lists HFCS as acceptable for those with FM. "HFCS is made up of almost half glucose and half fructose and may be absorbed just as well as sucrose (regular table sugar)"[7]. However, there are different types of HFCS:

> HFCS 90 (most commonly used in baked goods), approximately 90% fructose and 10% glucose
>
> HFCS 55 (most commonly used in soft drinks), approximately 55% fructose and 45% glucose
>
> HFCS 42 (most commonly used in sports drinks), approximately 42% fructose and 58% glucose [4]

As it is easy to see, only one of these falls within the 50% or less fructose limit. One problem is, foods containing HFCS do not state which HFCS it is, so we have no way of determining for sure if the glucose is greater than the fructose. The University of Virginia resource is the only one I have found which says HFCS is acceptable; all others warn against its use. My experience also indicates it is unacceptable for FM sufferers. A perusal of FM internet support sites has shown other FMer's also find it unacceptable.

Though controversial, many believe, and studies have shown, HFCS to be linked to various health problems including obesity, heart disease, and diabetes. According to the *Nutritional Research Center.Org,* "In 2005, if one looks at the actuarial curve on cardiovascular disease, obesity, hypoglycemia, and diabetes, they all parallel HFCS increase in the food chain — A FACT."

Think about it…in the mid '80s the health conscious movement began. Aerobics, working out at gyms, and other forms of exercise became the norm. The contradiction in these two facts tells me there is at least one major contributing factor. I believe it to be HFCS.

According to Satish Rao, M.D. of the University of Iowa, though we have long consumed fructose in the form of fruits, "…what has changed in recent decades is that many people in the United States eat vastly more fructose and in a purer form rather than mixed with other sugars." (HFCS) This leads me to the assumption that the super concentration of fructose I have been ingesting in the form of HFCS may have been detrimental to my health.

Once again, with HFCS, as with everything in this book, you must form your own opinion and make your own decisions.

Overweight and obesity

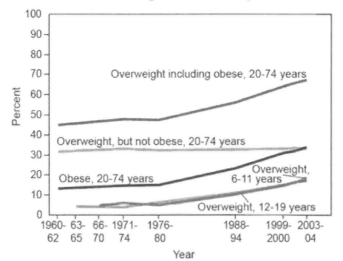

SOURCES: Centers for Disease Control and Prevention, National Center for Health Statistics, Health, United States, 2006 Figure 13. Data from the National Health and Nutrition Examination Survey.

According to the National Center for Health (NCH), average weight has increased, with obesity rates now at record levels. Between 1962 and 2000, obese people grew from 13% to 31% of the population. According to the NCH, one-third of U.S. adults, or over 72 million people, were obese in 2005-2006. Encarta Dictionary defines obese as having a body weight more than 20 percent greater than recommended for the relevant height.

What *Can* I Eat?

Good question. This is where the conflicting information really starts. One source will say a food is acceptable while another will say never eat it. For example, early on, my husband spent an entire afternoon comparing the six lists we had at that time for acceptable foods. Since I was still having problems despite a strict diet, he was hoping to discover a "for sure" list of foods I could eat. (See "Bob's List," (pg. 140) Of the six lists compared, there were five vegetables found on all six as acceptable. Of those five, my current research has shown at least two to be potentially unacceptable. So what is the FM sufferer to do?

First and foremost, educate yourself. Rather than writing a book of "dos and don'ts," we have tried to provide a source which will give you the reasoning behind the dos and don'ts, such as why to stay away from stone fruits (polyols) when sources say they are fine due to their fructose/glucose ratio. Hopefully, this will help you wade through some of the conflicting information.

It is recommended you begin with a sugar-free, fructose-free diet for a minimum of two weeks. This is the diet for HFI. Thankfully, it is not necessary to remain as strict as this diet requires. I stuck with it for about six weeks before beginning to add foods, in hopes of giving some extra relief to my taxed body. This amount of time was perhaps excessive, but if your symptoms are to the extreme point, as mine were, you may also wish to try extra time.

Adding foods must be done slowly, one at a time. The most difficult part of adding foods is, once you find a food which disagrees with you, you need to wait awhile, from several days to two weeks, to allow the body to return to normal before trying a new food. It is a very long process which takes a great deal of patience. I have not been very good with patience.

Food diaries are highly recommended. Current cited information may be helpful. Take care, as there is a great deal of misinformation available on the internet. The best thing is to know what to stay away from and why, then experiment with what is left (short list). Be patient; introduce foods one at a time. I have found two sources which tell me the fructose and glucose content on some foods: *http://www.nal.usda.gov/fnic/foodcomp/search/* and *http://www.nutritiondata.com/.* However, these sites still conflict with other information available during my research. I have used the above two sources to create one list, which is much easier to follow, specifically for the FMer. (See "Lists")

This cannot be said enough, read labels. An excellent example of the label being the FMer's friend is yogurt. Many popular yogurts have HFCS or at least corn syrup. Many organic varieties contain molasses or honey. All of these items are on the FMer's "no" list. But do not despair, safe yogurts do exist. We just have to look harder for them. Most will contain cane sugar; be sure you can handle small amounts before trying yogurt.

If you are accustomed to eating out frequently or eating boxed, frozen, or pre-prepared foods, you will need to be prepared to change. Learn to cook from scratch. Whole foods are not only healthier, but much easier for the FMer to discern acceptability than prepared foods. After all, there are no lists of ingredients to read and sort through.

Unfortunately, there are no "Safe for FM" labels required on foods…yet. Nor are nutrition labels required to divide the "sugars" into the types of sugars (fructose, glucose, sucrose, etc.), allowing us to determine the fructose/glucose ratio…yet. Perhaps as FM becomes more well known and the numbers of diagnosed FMer's increase, such labeling will be a reality. It was not long ago that we did not see "Gluten Free" on a label.

Ultimately, each FMer must customize their individual dict. Make your own lists of yes, no, and maybe foods. As and aid, we have provided various lists in the appendix of this book. Remember, these lists are not set in stone, add to them as you learn. Additionally, there may be foods which can only be eaten in combination with other foods or in small quantities. Remember, regardless if a list in this book or on a web-site says a certain food is okay, you cannot make the assumption it is okay for you until you are able to eat it symptom free on a consistent basis. Educate yourself and those around you. This is not an overnight process; it is a long-term experiment – and you are the lab rat.

Nutrition Notes

As stated earlier, I have long been a nutrition conscious person, especially with my children. I find it amusing that recently there has been a great deal of hype regarding colors of foods in our diets. It seems either the media or the health experts have just figured out that the greater the variety of natural colors in our diets, the more vitamins and minerals we will get, thus resulting in healthier bodies. By colors I refer to the dark green of spinach, Swiss chard or broccoli; the orange of carrots, oranges, or yams; the red of cherries, tomatoes or beets; the yellow of peaches, corn, or squash; the white of cauliflower, potatoes or onions, etc.

My children will tell you this is something I have stressed since they were small. As the old saying goes, "Variety is the spice of life." In my way of thinking, this refers to food. Unfortunately, this variety can be quite difficult for an FMer to achieve. Even when we can include a color, it is often necessary to restrict the quantity to such a small amount, we wonder how many benefits we are receiving. How, for instance, do we get the lycopene in tomatoes and other red fruits, which is believed to be so beneficial toward preventing cancer? (Though this was meant as a rhetorical question, I decided to include an answer...pink grapefruit.)

It has always been my opinion that if a person eats a good, nutritious diet, consisting of a wide variety of healthy foods, supplements should not be necessary. Unfortunately, few people these days seem to fit into this category. For the FMer, it is a near impossibility.

In addition to remaining conscious of the variety in my diet, we have begun taking a good quality multi-vitamin. This was also encouraged by my physician. Supplements with inulin and fructooligosaccaride (FOS), both types of fructans, should be avoided. (Inulin is also used to replace fat in low-fat foods, so beware.) Finding a good vitamin in either capsule form or gel-cap form without it being a "mega-vitamin" with an excessive percentage of nutrients is not easy.

I stress either capsule or gel-cap forms because I want to be getting the most for my money. A quick study will show most pill form vitamins are compressed so tightly they do not have time to absorb into your system before passing on to your bowels (gee, sounds vaguely familiar), thus wasting the remainder of the pill. If a pill does not completely dissolve within ten minutes in a glass of water, it will also not dissolve within your system.

Additionally, we take fish oil supplements, due to the increased fats in our diet since my diagnosis, to help assure they will not be clogging our arteries. The doctor has said this is a wise choice. The increased fats are an attempt to compensate for the lack of flavor, now that healthy things like onions and garlic are problematic. There are, of course, methods for reducing fats, especially bad fats, from our diets. Olive oil, a good fat, has become a staple in our household. Also, frying does not mean we have to use large quantities of oil. We often "dry fry" food, or fry it using just enough oil to coat the skillet. We will even wipe the excess oil with a paper towel to assure a *dry* fry.

Probiotics and prebiotics have been a source of controversy among the FM community. Some say they may help, some say they are a waste of money, and yet others say they will make matters worse (too much bacteria already, why add to the mix?). One FMer said her dietician said to stay away from anything with them.

My thoughts are, they should not hurt anything, so I take one per day; if part of my problem is SBBO, the probiotic may help conquer that problem. After all, part of the purpose of probiotics is for the good bacteria to kill the bad bacteria. Be aware, there are many different types of probiotics. One of them, the probiotic bacterium, *Lactobacillus plantarum* 299V, was found to be effective in reducing IBS symptoms.[10] Just be sure they do not contain inulins.

When I first began my research I thought probiotics and prebiotics were terms used interchangeably. I have since learned that probiotics are active mainly in the small intestine and prebiotics work only within the large intestine. When used in combination, they are referred to as synbiotics.

Recently, I have added vitamin D_3 to the mix of supplements I take. After being told my vitamin D levels are low, I did a bit of research into its source, its benefits, and what the effects of too little can be.

The most plentiful source of vitamin D is the sun (the USB's produce D_3). Regrettably, many of us spend the vast majority of each day indoors, we live in areas where the sun is in short supply during the winter months, or we live in smoggy areas. When we do get outside, we use sunscreen to prevent skin cancer; unfortunately the down side to increased use of sunscreen is, it also blocks the body from absorbing this necessary vitamin. Skin pigment also plays a roll in the amount of vitamin D absorbed by the skin; the darker the skin, the less easily the vitamin D absorbs.

Other sources are fish and fortified products, such as cereals and milk. The D vitamin obtained through food is D_2. Regrettably, it is difficult to acquire enough of this essential vitamin from food alone. See page 168 for a list of vitamin D sources.

Vitamin D deficiency can lead to or is associated with: autoimmune diseases such as multiple sclerosis and rheumatoid arthritis, diabetes, cardiovascular diseases, cancer, depression, fractures, high blood pressure, infectious diseases, muscle weakness, osteoporosis, and rickets. Pediatricians throughout the country have surprisingly been seeing patients suffering from rickets, which was once thought of as a problem from previous times. Furthermore, studies have shown that sufferers of chronic pain frequently have low levels of vitamin D. Sufferers of restless leg syndrome have reported improvement upon supplementation with vitamin D.

While there is some controversy surrounding the recommended allowance of vitamin D, there is no doubt we need to be sure we are not deficient in this essential vitamin. Rather than supplementing your diet "just-in-case," I suggest you ask your doctor to check your levels of vitamin D. This is done with a simple blood test.

When taking a supplement of a single vitamin or mineral, it is important to be sure you need it or are not taking excess amounts. The vitamins and minerals in our bodies are a delicate balance. If one vitamin or mineral is low, we show symptoms. This is examled by: with low vitamin D, we may have achy bones; with low vitamin C we may incur excessive bruising. On the other end of the spectrum, if we are taking levels which are too high, we can create an imbalance of other vitamins and minerals, causing other symptoms. Multi-vitamins are formulated to allow for this balance. Before taking any single vitamin or any mega vitamins, check with your doctor.

Remember also that it is important to list any vitamin, mineral, or herbal supplements on your list of medications taken when seeing your physician. Certain combinations of medications and supplements are inadvisable due to interactions, being rendered ineffective by their combination, or potential false results on tests. Also, before a planned surgery, certain supplements need to be discontinued due to potential adverse effects.

Ultimately, FMer's must be extra conscious of the nutritional value of their diets. I have found this to be something I must do on my own since I have been unable to locate a dietician who is familiar enough with FM to be of assistance; we live in a remote, small town. I still attempt to vary the color of my meals as much as possible, adding the supplements mentioned above. Though I may not be achieving the nutritional value I hope to, my body is obviously healthier and happier with this new eating lifestyle as evidenced by a reduction and/or elimination of symptoms previously mentioned.

Mourning

If you have been diagnosed with FM, it is important to recognize that you have suffered a loss, one which will change most people's lives dramatically. Your loved ones will also need to understand this. As with any major loss in life, you will go through a mourning period. *Let yourself mourn.* You have, in a sense, suffered a death; the death of a way of life, a way of eating, a way of socializing.

Allowing yourself to mourn does not mean giving in to the depression, anger, or denial you may be experiencing, but instead, being aware of it for what it is and realizing it is something you *can* get though.

As with mourning anything, there is a process with stages. Familiarizing yourself with these stages may help you to understand and therefore better cope with the process. I must emphasize, this too shall pass. You *can* get used to FM. You *can* learn how to eat. You *can* learn to accept your condition. You can even learn to handle food in social situations.

St*eps of Mourning*

1. Shock – This is rather self describing. It is shocking to discover the "healthy" eating you have been doing is actually contributing to making you ill. It is shocking to learn how many foods you can no longer eat. It is shocking to learn what is included in so many foods you eat.

2. Denial – Your denial may be in the form of eating freely, which will result in a harsh reminder you are unable to do this. Or you may deny the permanency of this condition (I still have hope). You may even choose to hide your condition from friends or family to avoid such things as questions, pity, and disbelief.

3. Anger – It is easy to get angry about this. Anger and denial seem to accompany each other frequently during this process for FMer's. There is so much to be angry about, but there is also so much for which

to be thankful. Try to focus on these.
Early after my diagnosis, when I was quite
angry and busy feeling sorry for myself, I
realized I actually had it quite easy. I
currently work with three people who are
battling cancer. For them, it is life or
death. For them, treatment is agonizing.
For them, merely having to restrict their
diet would be a relief. How dare I spend
so much time and energy wallowing in
self-pity? I was, and still am, ashamed of
myself for this. When I begin to feel sorry
for myself I try to remember my co-
workers and others who have *real*
problems.

4. Depression – Anger has a way of leading
   to self-pity, this in turn contributes to
   depression. To help you deal with
   depression see the chapter on depression
   and seek professional help if needed

5. Acceptance – I am finally, after two years,
   at this point. Do I still have to deal with
   any of the aforementioned steps? You bet

I do. I still get angry. I still wallow in self-pity and depression. I'm constantly testing the boundaries. I even still try denial at times (like during our recent Thanksgiving dinner, for which I paid the price). But I deal with these less and less all the time. You too, will reach this point. Unlike mourning the loss of a loved one, when acceptance brings its own mini-mourning due to the guilt which accompanies it, there is a certain pride in reaching this point in this mourning process for an FMer. Though we are unable to conquer the condition, we can overcome the mental, emotional, and physical effects of it. Thus, we win!

These steps may come as listed in the order given, or not; or in any combination. You may skip a step or two. Awareness will be your key to "successful mourning." What is successfully mourning? Not falling into the depths of depression, not driving your friends and family away, and finding ways to accept and live with this problem while still feeling like you have a full life are some of the signs of successful mourning.   In other words, learning to accept and deal with your new life is successful mourning.

Additional Information

"It is believed that up to 36% of the European population has fructose malabsorption in a more or less severe form, and approximately one-half of affected individuals are symptomatic"[5]. This figure is estimated to be far higher in the United States (could this be related to the extensive additives in our foods, such as HFCS, which is rarely used outside the U.S?). Unfortunately, it is a little-known condition, even among the medical community, resulting in frequent lack of proper diagnosis.

Another result of this lack of familiarity with FM is the general public, acquaintances, friends, family, and even some medical personnel may respond to the FMer's diagnosis with doubt. It sounds so odd and unhealthy, people often have difficulty grasping that it is a genuine condition which deserves respect.

In a survey of 33 Oregon family physicians, internists, and nurse practitioners which I initiated while researching this book, of the twelve who responded, only four respondents were even vaguely familiar with FM, with the same number being familiar with breath hydrogen testing (not necessarily the same ones). *None were familiar with breath hydrogen testing for FM, which must be done specifically for fructose.* Surprisingly, after doing the survey, there were two respondents who said they "may" be inclined to familiarize themselves with FM and one who said "no" to familiarization. Thankfully, the remaining respondents indicated they would definitely be familiarizing themselves with FM. My question is, why would any primary heath care provider not want to familiarize themselves with FM?

The importance of primary care physicians being knowledgeable of FM becomes obvious when one considers that many believe *irritable bowel syndrome* (IBS) to be a catch-all for an unexplained group of symptoms, not a diagnosis. By definition, a syndrome is not a diagnosis but a group of recognized symptoms. Encarta Dictionary defines syndrome as "1. group of identifying signs and symptoms, 2. things that form pattern." It is estimated as many as

45-75% of those "diagnosed" with IBS actually have FM. Others may have lactose intolerance, gluten intolerance, or yeast intolerance. Proper testing is essential. What if I had accepted prescription laxatives without question? Many other symptoms would likely have continued without "treatment."

The depression associated with FM is thought to have a connection with the folic acid which is also associated with FM. Clinical trials have shown, of those who tested positive for FM, average folic acid levels were lower than normal, "Folic acid deficiency may contribute to the development of mental depression"[5]. (See the chapter on depression.) While low folic acid levels are associated with cardiovascular disease and neural-tube defects in newborns, "folic acid supplementation was found to reduce the relative risk for the development of colon carcinoma (cancer). These findings suggest that fructose malabsorption could be a risk factor in the development of these diseases"[5].

The systemic inflammation associated with FM is also believed to have detrimental long-term effects. Joint pain, allergies, heart attack, stroke, and premature aging are a few of the possible conditions associated with inflammation.

These findings help to support my theory that anything which causes such a vast array of symptoms must have some associated long-term effects, which is dramatically opposed to the information I was given upon diagnosis-that there are no long term effects of FM. This is one more reason primary care providers should familiarize themselves with FM.

Often coupled with FM is small bowel bacterial overgrowth (SBBO), which is exactly what it sounds like. The bacteria in the small intestine have multiplied to extra large quantities, which cause symptoms similar to FM. However, SBBO can*not* be diagnosed with a breath hydrogen test, so if your breath hydrogen test shows you to have FM, it is not SBBO, though you could have SBBO in combination with FM. While SBBO can be treated with antibiotics, the two conditions seem to be interdependent, thus requiring repeated or long term use of antibiotics. Due to the negative aspects of long-term antibiotic use, this is ill-advised. Having been on antibiotics long term several years ago while fighting an infection, I have, in fact, theorized the possibility that antibiotics may have been a contributing factor in causing my enterocytes to stop functioning properly, thus being one possible cause of my FM. In my research on the internet, many FMer's state they have also taken high dosage or long-term antibiotics.

Causes of Fructose Malabsorption

Unfortunately, the exact cause of FM is unknown. Most researchers theorize it is caused by the excessive amounts of fructose which we consume in today's society. One trip through the grocery store to read labels will leave a person asking why everything we eat must have some form of sugar, especially HFCS.

Another theory is the overuse of antibiotics. Unfortunately, antibiotics are non-discriminatory. Though they can do a great job of killing the bad bacteria which make us sick, they are also busy attacking and destroying good bacteria. The body is a delicate balance of bacteria, yeast, and other beastly things. By reducing the good bacteria in our bodies through the use of antibiotics, we throw that balance off. This is why a bacterial infection is often followed by a yeast infection. I wonder…what is to keep these often-time strong drugs (antibiotics), which we may also be getting from their overuse in our meats and dairy, from destroying other essential body elements such as enzymes and enterocytes?

Some wonder if it could be hereditary. While we must reiterate that FM must not be confused with Hereditary Fructose Intolerance (HFI), this does not mean FM could not also be hereditary. A little time spent on any support group site can reveal this possibility. If it were not hereditary or at least predisposed in families, why do we see families with several members who have FM?

Just as genetic makeup predisposes some people to obesity, alcoholism, and diabetes, perhaps our genetic may increase the likelihood of FM in our families. To follow this a bit further, just as with obesity, alcoholism, or diabetes, perhaps a careful diet for those predisposed to FM may help to prevent it.

Yet another theory is the extensive use of pesticides, herbicides, and other alterations to our foods. If these processes are meant to kill organisms, what is to keep them from killing the organisms and delicate body parts we all need to function normally? Almost every food we eat has been sprayed with something, or several things, and/or altered in some manner.   In fact, the more you think about it, the more frightening it becomes.

Dietary Changes – Going Organic

While considering the potential destructive effects of pesticides, herbicides, dyes, and other alterations (all of this I call "ized") to our foods, we realized we had both been considering "going organic" for years, but we were both too cheap to convince ourselves to do it. Face it, organic is more expensive. After much discussion and mental financial tug-of-war, we determined it was time to go organic. Why would two professed cheapskates make a decision which would effectively double their food bill?

Consider milk. By buying organic fat free milk we usually pay the same for a half gallon that we used to pay for a full gallon of non-organic milk. This seems insane until you consider what has gone into that **non**-organic gallon of milk. Besides probably being a genetically altered animal, chances are, the feed the cow eats has been altered, "ized," or contains animal bi-products. The cow has probably been shot full of hormones, antibiotics, and other medications to help it grow, produce more, and stay healthy despite not being free to exercise and being fed a diet unnatural to cows. After the cow is milked, the milk undergoes processing. Consequently, the regular milk we drink has at least a triple "izing" to it: feed, cow, milk. To me, that just does not sound healthy. Don't forget, this includes milk products like cheese, ice cream, and sour cream.

Milk examples only one food. Read a few labels. Do a bit of math. Add all the artificial additives, chemicals, dyes, irradiation, hormones, antibiotics, etc. you get in all the different foods you consume and you may be eating the equivalent of a full meal, or at least a snack, each day of nothing but "izings." Then add to this the products we put on our skin. Medication patches work so well because the skin readily absorbs what is on it. The point is…how many artificial additives can we consume before our bodies begin to be affected by them?

With proper nutrition being a concern, the fact that "75 published studies have found that organic food is more nutritious than nonorganic,"[12] is just one more reason to take a closer look at organics. This means the vitamin and mineral levels of organics foods have shown to be higher than those of non-organic foods. Though I can not help but think they would have to be more nutritious when they are not full of poisons.

We have found ways to reduce the financial impact of going organic. We shop at Grocery Outlet, an outlet store in the West for groceries, and they now carry a variety of organic products. Unfortunately, being an outlet store, the products come and go. We stock up when we find products we like. We watch the other stores for sales on organics; most stores now have at least a small organic section. We have also found a couple of direct sources for organics in the form of local growers. You may be able to find organic growers at your local farmers market. If you are fortunate enough to live in a city with grocers who specialize in organic and natural foods, the search for organics will be much easier for you.

Growing your own is also an option. Even apartment dwellers can plant window gardens. Though we are not yet growing our own, we are planning a greenhouse so we will soon have homegrown organic produce. This is one more way we can take control in what sometimes seems an out-of-control condition.

If all-organic is budget-prohibitive, you may want to restrict organic purchases to those having the greatest impact. When buying organic, choose thin-skinned or no skin item, such as milk, eggs, celery, mushrooms, zucchini, etc. Then you can buy non-organic thick-skinned items: oranges, bananas, pomegranates, nuts, etc. If you choose to do this, keep in mind that these foods can also take in poisons just like they take in water, so this is a compromise.

According to the definition provided by the National e-Commerce Extension Initiative at http://srdc.msstate.edu/ecommerce/curricula/farm_mg mt/glossary.htm "To be labeled organic, all fresh or processed foods sold in the United States, including imports, must be produced according to the national organic standards and certified by an inspection agency accredited by the USDA. Before their crops can be certified, all organic farmers must use only approved materials. They must develop an organic farm management plan, keep detailed records, and be inspected annually by an accredited certification agency. All companies that manufacture organic food products must follow similar strict requirements." This definition agrees with those provided by other sites. The Organic Trade Association's website at http://www.ota.com/organic/faq.html provides an excellent source for information regarding organic products.

A few words on "natural," it has no meaning on anything but meat. There are no guidelines or regulations guiding or limiting its use. There are a few "natural" products we use, but we have also researched into these products to discover exactly what their use of the word "natural" means. For meat, the USDA requires products to be free of artificial ingredients, colorings, preservatives, and unnecessary processing. We purchase a local "natural" beef. Our research has shown it to be locally raised, in pastures, eating the untreated grass grown in those pastures, without being forced to consume corn (our research has taught us that "corn fed" is not a good thing, cows are not designed to consume corn and it makes them sick without the use of antibiotics), using no growth hormones, antibiotics, or other artificial enhancements. While this beef does not have the "certified organic" label, it has been grown and produced in essentially the same manner as organic beef, the grower has simply decided against the expense of certification. Additionally, it may mean the pastures on which the cow is fed have not gone an appropriate amount of time without prohibited substances to be certified or it is too near areas which use chemicals to be certified organic.

From the FM standpoint, I never need to worry about HFCS being used in organic products. HFCS may be made from corn, but it is *not* organic. This allows me to be able to eat some snacks and packaged products I would not be able to consume in non-organic foods. Unfortunately, organic does not mean I can stop reading labels. I still need to verify the product does not contain one of the many foods I am unable to eat. But it does make it easier to find products such as cereals, dressings, and snacks.

Another thing we have noticed since beginning the switch to organics. It tastes better. For example, the milk we discussed earlier, we have noticed a subtle, yet distinctly different taste from "regular" milk. Recently it dawned on me why our milk had been so "dull" the last few days; I had picked up a half-gallon of milk at a store which did not have organic milk, meaning I had to buy the non-organic brand. Even I was surprised with the revelation. Meat is also different. If you are over the age of 40 you may remember meat having more flavor, marbling, and color. When you buy organic, it still does. Tomatoes...okay, FMer's can't even think about eating them anyway, but our families can and they deserve a wonderful, red, juicy, flavorful fruit; not the anemic looking, woody textured, flavorless imitator we see today. (Hint: fried green tomatoes in small quantities do not seem to bother me – see recipe section.)

There have been aspects to going organic which have surprised me. When I make a meal or send lunch to school with our daughter or my husband knowing it is all-organic, there is a sense of relief, coupled with pride. By combining sound nutrition with organic food, I know I am providing my family the healthiest meals I possibly can. This is especially important to me due to the concern about lack of variety FM has caused in our lives.

Going organic has given me back some of the control I lost when diagnosed. In addition to mourning the loss of food as I knew it, depression for me was aggravated by the loss of control. FM became the controller of my diet; food choices were no longer mine. Now, when I find a food I can eat which seems to defy the restrictions, I have accomplished something, I have taken back some control. Organic has given me something to focus on other than what I am unable eat. It has put a positive element of eating back into my life. It has empowered me. Organic is my version of "making lemonade out of lemons."

Additionally, shopping is not nearly as depressing when buying organic. Without the constant threat of HFCS, there are far more options open to me. Though we live in a small town, when we get to a city with one of those wonderful food stores which specialize in organic foods, it is empowering to be able to walk down every isle of the store and know I can find things I can eat. Living in a small town, finding organics is a challenge, but I love a good challenge.

When visiting my daughter's family in Maryland during the birth of our grandson, they seemed quite unflustered by my eating restrictions. They cook from scratch anyway and use primarily organic foods.

If you still are not convinced that going organic may help your with your FM struggles, perhaps you will respond to the "green" argument. Organic farming is much friendlier to the environment. Non-organic farming uses tremendous quantities of herbicides, pesticides, and chemical fertilizers, which are not only on the food we eat but also make their way into our lakes, rivers, oceans, and even the underground water. Of course, this can also affect wildlife, such as the fish and seafood we consume. Surely, if we are willing to absorb the extra costs for other green products, we will be more than willing to do so with the food we consume?

Eating Out

As much as I would like to conclude this section with one word..."don't," this is not a realistic solution. The challenge of eating out with FM is one which must be mastered by each FMer in a way which best suits the individual. It is not easy. Your companions may find it embarrassing or annoying. Restaurants are problematic in that you never know what the ingredients are. I have found the nicer the restaurant, the more difficult it is to eat pain-free. Think about it, onions and garlic are used extensively in cooking, the fancier the restaurant, the more in love with onions the chef will be. Though I really can't blame chefs, onions add flavor!

For the sake of your health and well-being, speak up. This applies whether deciding on a restaurant or choosing from the menu. Never be shy about explaining you are very restricted in what you can eat. I have even begun saying I have allergies rather than a restricted diet due to the problem of servers thinking I am "dieting" to lose weight, thus being somewhat unimportant. While FM is not technically allergies, I need them to understand the importance of my many requests. Being excessively honest, this was very difficult for me at first, then a co-worker pointed out, it does make me sick, just not vomit sick, so I should not feel guilty. After reviewing my own list of symptoms, I agree, it does make me sick.

Speak up! On a recent business trip with co-workers I requested we not go to the Mexican restaurant which had been suggested. It is simply too difficult to find acceptable food on the Mexican menu, especially in an authentic Mexican restaurant. On the other hand, Taco Bell is one of the few "restaurants" I can count on. It is not that I can eat a lot on the menu, rather that there is one item I know I can eat, a soft taco. Besides not causing me to react, it has the extra added advantage of being cheap...excuse me...a great bargain.

Chinese food; once again, this is a problematic area. Let me preface this by noting that Chinese (the American version) has long been my favorite food. I must point out a few notable aspects regarding Chinese food. Because I enjoy it, I have a tendency to overeat, which is one of the "triggers" for FM sufferers. If I eat it as served, I will be doubled over before I finish my meal, so I don't need to overeat to "enjoy" the repercussions. By ordering my meal without MSG, I can delay or lessen the onset of symptoms. The only sure way I have found to eat Chinese symptom-free is to order carefully and ask that all items be steamed. I order a lunch dish served at my local restaurant and request it all be steamed only – hold the carrots and onions, resulting in a plate of steamed rice (I can add soy sauce to it-though not all FMer's can handle soy sauce), steamed broccoli, and steamed shrimp. I must admit, I occasionally give in and make a conscious decision to eat anything I want, and later ask my husband to never let me do that again.

Steak houses; be careful. I have found this to be an easy place to eat if I am very specific. For example, ask for the steak to be cooked with only salt and pepper, since the rubs used in some steak houses can contain a lot of pain. If you are planning to eat seafood, be cautious. Don't hesitate to request it be cooked without their sauces and rubs. Choose the baked potato. Mashed potatoes frequently contain garlic and other forbidden items and rice pilaf most assuredly contains onions and probably some veggies which are unacceptable. Speaking of veggies, be sure to ask what kind they are serving. Request steamed or grilled without extra flavorings if possible. Dessert, stay away from it. Unless you are in a very high-end restaurant, that luscious looking cheesecake was probably purchased frozen and invariably includes HFCS.

Pastas in white sauce, such as alfredo, sound safe until you realize the chance is probably 100% the chef used onions at some point in making the sauce. This renders Italian to be difficult also, though not impossible. The key is to go to a restaurant which makes each dish as it is ordered and request offending items to be left out. For obvious reasons, any tomato saucy item is unacceptable. If you order pizza, request ranch dressing or a garlic ranch (if you can tolerate a small amount of garlic) sauce to be used in place of tomato pizza sauce. This is not fool proof.

The majority of dressings have HFSC and garlic can be problematic and may contain onions. Pizza is one of those things I hope for the best and expect the worst. Additionally, toppings for an FMer are limited. Remember processed meats, such as Canadian bacon, bacon, pepperoni, and sausage, are out; so meat choices are quite limited. Chicken and beef are possibilities. Mushrooms, bean sprouts, spinach, zucchini, bell peppers, and hot peppers are some possibilities in the way of vegetables. Then, of course, there is cheese. Remember, pizza provides an excellent opportunity to make your own, using safe ingredients.

Though I would love to be able to say what you can order in any given restaurant, we are so limited on restaurants in our small town that I lack the experience needed to do so. What I can recommend, and probably more useful in the long run, are some general guidelines.

- Salads: Either pick out items like onions, cucumbers, tomatoes, etc, and set aside/give away. Or simply request these items be left off the salad.

- Salad dressing: Learn to enjoy salad without it, ask for a lemon wedge on the side to squeeze on the salad, stick with oil and vinegar, or have a small container of an acceptable organic or homemade dressing of your choice in your purse or pocket.

- Meats: Request no extra sauces be added.

- Gravy: Be cautious, ask if they make it in-house, many restaurants use gravy mixes or canned which probably contain HFCS, especially brown gravy.

- French Fries: These can lead to confusion. They should be safe to eat, however not all French fries are "real." Some are mashed potatoes with other stuff mixed in, like onion powder, which have been formed into fries. The other problem is the type of oil used. I tend to note which place's fries cause me problems and which don't.

- Try to order foods as basic as possible. Plain steak, plain veggies, baked potato, etc.

- Know the menu before going; it saves time, frustration, and the possibility of needing to leave without eating. Many restaurants list their menus on the internet or in the phone book. If necessary, get a copy of the menu from the restaurant before going.

- Don't be afraid to ask if an item contains HFCS or onions. The server may need to ask the chef or read the label.

- Avoid rush hours in restaurants. This allows the server to give more individualized service and the chef time to make exceptions.

- Breakfasts are usually easier to order.

- Eggs and omelets are usually safe, though be cautious of the ingredients in the omelet. It will probably require holds/adds.

- Breakfast fried potatoes often contain onions, be sure to ask or stick with hash browns. Though it may be wise to verify they don't add onions to their hash browns and that they are fresh, not frozen. Many frozen hash browns contain unsafe ingredients.

- If you are aching for pancakes, you might try taking a small container of organic berry jelly with you to serve as topping in place of syrup. Then remember quantity is important and have only one pancake with a very small amount of jelly. If possible, choose buckwheat pancakes. Despite the name, buckwheat is not wheat and is acceptable.

- Avoid cured meats such as bacon since they are often cured with honey or molasses.

- Avoid processed meats such as sausage, they frequently contain or may be cured with unacceptable ingredients.

- Most commercial breads contain HFCS so ordering toast is risky. Sometimes sourdough is free of HFCS, but not always. Biscuits are sometimes an option, especially if they are homemade, not packaged.

- When ordering fish and chips, request no tarter sauce (I have a tendency to forget and use it). My friend from England taught me how to eat fish as the English do, with malt vinegar instead of tarter sauce.

- Avoid soups; chances are very good they contain onions.

- Place a roll of Smarties® or glucose tablets next to your plate, eating one occasionally to help guard against any hidden fructose. Remember, this can backfire if the food contains fructans, such as onions.

Gatherings, such as employee dinners and receptions, pose another problem. Being catered, the foods should all be labeled "dangerous for FMer's." We have decided the best way for me to deal with these situations is to eat before going and then chose (if a buffet) the closest things to "safe" I see. At a recent luncheon I chose a very small amount of Caesar salad and some homemade bread (the caterer's specialty) and hoped for the best. I would have stepped out during the lunch portion of the meeting, but it was a working lunch, so a discrete exit was not an option.

Help for the Hurting

What to do to stop the symptoms caused by FM is a big question. The most obvious answer being…stop consuming things which cause problems. This, obviously, would be a statement made by a non-FMer.

If you know or suspect you will be eating something you should not eat, take a dextrose (glucose) tablet before eating to help correct the fructose/glucose ratio. If you cannot find these, in a pinch the candy, *Smarties®,* may be of assistance. These sweet little candies first ingredient is dextrose. Even better, there is no HFCS. Of course, they are not organic, containing much in the way of food dyes. Also, one little roll contains a whopping 100 calories. Be aware, these will **not** help with fructans; in fact, they may exacerbate the problem with fructans. If I suspect a food item may have an unfavorable ratio, I will eat a few *Smarties®.* While eating out at a recent dinner theater, I kept a roll next to my charger (the bottom plate which remains throughout the meal), eating a few with each course. This even got me through a small glass of Merlot and the establishment's marvelous, signature, grape salad. It may have added an extra 100 calories, but it made my evening far more pleasant.

Unfortunately, it seems regardless how careful the FMer is with diet, something sneaks its way in and we find ourselves in pain, full of gas, dashing to the bathroom, with bile in our throats, feeling like a balloon, battling a headache, or just feeling crappy and lethargic. Now what?

There are ways to battle the symptoms which otherwise seem to defy the typical remedies. Listed below are some things which have helped me. Unfortunately, some symptoms, like ballooning, I simply have to allow time to pass. Thankfully I have been able to take a more pro-active approach to others.

Rice bag...If you are not familiar with these, you are in for a treat. They are the microwave-age version of a hot water bottle. Typically it is a cloth envelope of various shapes and sizes which is filled with rice, flax, corn, or wheat. The one I use most is filled with flax and rice. It can be heated in the microwave for warmth or left in the freezer for a cold compress. You can make it yourself or purchase one in stores, on the internet, or at craft fairs. They are quite simple to make with instructions readily available on the internet. Some also have added ingredients such as lavender or cinnamon for aromatherapy purposes or simply to smell good. I have several of these in various sizes for different uses which I keep in the freezer and available to pop in the microwave. I even have a pair of rice bag booties for those times when I am unable to sleep because my feet are cold

Stomach pain – heated rice bag on tummy, drink water. Be careful not to overheat the rice bag, it can cause burns.

Headache – frozen rice bag on head, ibuprofen, drink water, hot shower (the steam helps open swollen sinus passages and it is relaxing).

Migraine – whatever it takes!

Acid indigestion or bile in throat – baking soda, be sure to follow the directions on the box or they can be found at http://www.armhammer.com/basics/magic/#12 , soda crackers, I use organic since many non-organic ones contain HFCS.

Gas – heated rice bag, drink water, exercise. Unfortunately I have not found simethecone or any of the usual anti-gas products helpful.

Puffiness (balloon-like) – wait it out. I try drinking extra water in the hope it will help to flush whatever is puffing me. If you have found a remedy to help with this, please let me know. Ibuprofen or a similar anti-inflammatory may be of some help.

Constipation – Myralax (check with your doctor first), water, interesting reading material.

Diarrhea – While this is not an area in which I have experience (check with your doctor), my research does show you should be very conscious of remaining hydrated. Drink plenty of water. For excessive diarrhea, you may want to try something which will replace electrolytes, such as Gatorade (if you can tolerate this), but be sure to read labels, some Gatorade contains HFCS.

Unfortunately, while researching to try to find help for those of you with this problem, I discovered most of the "cures" are items FMer's must avoid. If you have other remedies not listed here, please let me know and I will include them in future editions to aid to our fellow FMer's.

Because I am obviously not an attorney, I would suggest you consult one before pursuing the following. If you have been challenged by problems on the job due to the effects of FM, it is my understanding that FM is covered by the American's with Disabilities Act (ADA). As a payroll specialist, I recently read about a Supreme Court decision which allowed that an employee with bowel/bladder problems must be relieved from duty to attend to bodily needs regardless of break periods (unsure of the source). Also, the ADA Amendments Act of 2008, which took effect January 2009, now specifies a list of *major life activities*, including major bodily functions such as bowel and bladder, as covered by the ADA. For those of you with diarrhea reactions, this could allow you to run to the much-needed bathroom, despite it not being break-time. For those of us with constipation problems, this may provide protection when we get "stuck" on the toilet and exceed our break or arrive late to work.

Depression

Due to the relationship between FM and depression, as well as the likelihood of an onset of depression after a diagnosis of FM, we feel the inclusion of a chapter about depression essential to the completeness of this book. Most of this chapter is an adaptation of two papers I wrote on the subject. As a result, it may include more information than is necessary for the scope of FM, but since many FMer's may have been fighting depression for extended periods of time, we did not edit it as much as we could have.

Why is depression associated with FM? The unabsorbed fructose which has passed on to an FMer's lower intestine then bonds with tryptophan, thus rendering the tryptophan unabsorbable. Tryptophan is an amino acid needed to make serotonin, which helps guard against depression. Some call it a happy neurotransmitter. Plus, tryptophan becomes melatonin, which is the substance in us telling us to sleep when it becomes dark. Thus, FMer's have problems sleeping, and lack of sleep contributes to depression. Is it just me, or is there is a pattern forming here? On the brighter side...when we stop consuming fructose, we start producing tryptophan so the depression goes away or at least improves.

Foods high in tryptophan include shrimp, sesame seed, and milk. For a more complete listing, see the list beginning on page 170. Also available are supplements, though as always, caution should be used in this area,. In 1989, an outbreak of an auto-immune illness called eosinophilia-myalgia syndrome (EMS) was attributed to L-tryptophan, resulting in the ban of this supplement in the United States. The problem was ultimately traced to one manufacturer in Japan. In 2002, the FDA removed their ban on its sale. Remember, FMer's do not need to supplement, they simply need to stop consuming fructose so the tryptophan can absorb.

There are other factors which affect the absorption of tryptophan. Vitamin B6 is also necessary for the conversion of tryptophan to serotonin, thus a deficiency in B6 may also contribute to depression. B6 can be found in bananas, salmon, turkey, spinach, and hazelnuts, to name a few. Additionally, there are conditions and life style choices which can reduce the conversion of tryptophan to serotonin: smoking, high sugar intake, alcohol abuse, excessive consumption of protein, hypoglycemia, and diabetes. As always, be sure to have your physician check your B6 levels and determine a dosage before beginning any supplements.

According to the National Institute of Mental Health, 9.5% of the population of the United States suffers from depression in any given year. Yet, depression remains vastly misunderstood, the butt of jokes, ridicule, and disbelief. It is referred to by some as an excuse for laziness. Although the long list of famous sufferers includes Abraham Lincoln, Samuel Clemens, Sergey Rachmaninoff, Irving Berlin, Walt Whitman, and Vincent van Gogh; acceptance of victims has been slow.

As a survivor of clinical depression, I know the embarrassment, reality, pain, and disruption of depression firsthand. During my initial bout with major depression, I had no idea what it was and feared I was going insane. By my second episode I knew what it was and sought to educate myself further, as well as received extensive treatment. However, the embarrassment of a mental disorder limited my circle of confidants regarding my condition and treatment to three people. Years later, with maturity and good health, I determined never to keep silent regarding this subject again. If my experience or knowledge could help others, I must share it.

Depression, a mood disorder, has many degrees of severity ranging from mild "blues" of short duration to psychotic depression. The three major types of depression are bi-polar disorder, dysthymia, and major depressive disorder (also known as clinical depression).

Seasonal affective disorder (SAD), also known as winter depression, is a mild form of depression characterized by symptoms only during the winter. While SAD is almost unknown in tropical locations, it can be quite common in locations with extended winter, darkness, and rain. When coupled with another form of depression, this can result in an extreme depressive period.

Dysthymia is chronic, low level depression. During a life crisis, the sufferer may develop major depressive disorder, not in place of, but in addition to dysthymia.

Reactive depression, also known as adjustment disorder with depressed mood, is depression brought on as the result of an occurrence, such as the death of a loved one or the loss of a job. This is a category of last resort, used only if the depression does not fit another term.

Major depressive disorder is an overwhelming depression with many symptoms. Some of these symptoms seem inconsistent with the term "depression," and will be discussed in detail later in this chapter.

Melancholic depression, according to the Diagnostic and Statistical Manual of Mental Disorders (DSM-IV) is a state of complete anhedonia, the inability to experience pleasures.

Psychotic depression is characterized by delusions and hallucinations. This is an extremely severe depression which can result from untreated depression of other forms.

Bi-polar depression (or disorder) is characterized by episodes of depression followed by episodes of manic behavior, characterized by euphoria, inflated self-esteem, and temporary loss of reality. Though a mood disorder within the depression spectrum, it is considered a separate disorder and is treated differently than depression.

Major depressive disorder affects different people differently. While one person may have trouble eating or sleeping, another may eat and sleep excessively. Fidgeting, hand wringing, and pacing may highlight one person's movements, while slowed speech, reaction time, and body movements mark another person's movements. Some people have many symptoms of depression, others have only a few. For some, it is obvious they are sufferers of depression; while for others, day-to-day functions may be relatively unimpaired.

In addition to the often mentioned overwhelming sadness, despair, hopelessness, and loss of ability to experience pleasure, there are less publicized symptoms of depression. Overreaction to minor occurrences, inability to make decisions, inability to concentrate and remember, anger, and unexplained aches and pains are notable in sufferers. The inability to do basic things such as: get out of bed, clean house, bathe, or fix a meal is an often misunderstood symptom of depression. This inability is not laziness or a choice; it can be as debilitating as a broken leg is to walking.

Symptoms of depression are many, varying by severity of the depressed state and individual. The symptoms may last for weeks, months, or years. The following list is not to be considered all-inclusive, nor is an individual likely to experience all of them.

Concentration Problems

Easy Loss of Temper

Difficulties Making Decisions

Social Withdrawal

No Desire for Pleasurable Activities

Lack of Appetite

Increased Appetite

Excessive Sleeping

Insomnia

Restlessness

Excessive Crying

Decreased Energy

Thoughts of Death or Suicide

Increased Irritability

Difficulty Remembering

Difficulty Making Decisions

Lack of Motivation

Chronic Fatigue

Apathy

Complaining

Neglect of Personal Appearance

Persistent physical symptoms which do not respond to treatment, such as: headaches, digestive disorders, and chronic pain - could this be a result of FM?

Feelings of: sadness, emptiness, hopelessness, dysphoria, guilt, worthlessness, and pessimism

With typical depression, the patient will eat and sleep less; while atypical depression is characterized by oversleeping, overeating, and resulting rapid weight gain. This is usually the type I fight. I seldom do anything in the "typical" manner.

The diagnosis of depression should be made by a qualified professional such as a psychologist or psychiatrist. A review of all medications, including herbal remedies, over-the-counters drugs, alcohol, and illegal drugs should be included. Additionally, a medical examination is called for if there are physical symptoms present. Perhaps, with what we now know about FM, a breath hydrogen test should be standard.

Depression is highly responsive to treatment, which takes two forms, psychotherapy and medications. For mild to moderate depression, psychotherapy is the most appropriate, while more severe cases usually require medication with therapy. Recovery rates have been shown to be significantly higher when psychotherapy and drug therapy are used in combination. Medication relieves the physical symptoms, which allows the user to concentrate on psychotherapy, which teaches coping skills.

Helping the patient gain insights into the causes of depression, psychotherapy takes two forms. Interpersonal therapy focuses on managing relationships which cause and exacerbate depression.

Cognitive, also known as behavioral, therapy works to change negative thinking and behavior associated with depression. After significant improvement, therapists may use psychodynamic therapy, which focuses on resolving patient's conflicted feelings.

It is important to remember that therapists differ in ability just as any doctor, mechanic, accountant, or teacher does. If the therapy is not beneficial or if there is poor therapist/patient rapport, a new therapist should be sought, just as one would do if their mechanic's work was ineffective.

Drug therapy is a useful and necessary form of treatment for depression and should be used only in conjunction with psychotherapy. While medications allow for quick symptomatic relief, much like cold medications, they do not treat the disease. There are three basic forms of medications for the treatment of depression, none of which are habit forming, though stopping the medication must be done slowly to prevent reoccurrence of symptoms. Depression medications are not specd, a happy pill, or a substitute for therapy. Additionally, sedatives are not anti-depressants.

The three forms of anti-depressants are tricyclics, selective serotonin reuptake inhibitors (SSRI's), and monoamine oxidase inhibitors (MAOI's). Each type has its own uses as well as side affects. The type of depression helps to determine which medication type will be effective.

Tricyclics are an older form of anti-depressant. Potential side effects may be: dry mouth, constipation, bladder problems, sexual problems, blurred vision, dizziness, and drowsiness in the daytime. While few users suffer all or even several of these symptoms, most usually disappear after adjusting to the medication.

Selective serotonin reuptake inhibitors (SSRI's) are one of the new medications for depression and affect neurotransmitters such as dopamine or norepinephrine. They have fewer side effects than tricyclics; headache, nausea, nervousness, insomnia, agitation, and sexual problems may plague the user.

While these same side effects apply to monoamine oxidase inhibitors (MAOI's), the other new class of medications used to treat depression, additional precautions must be taken to avoid foods and drugs with high levels of tyramine, which could result in a hypertensive crisis, leading to stroke. These foods include cheese, wine, and pickles, as well as decongestants.

All anti-depressants must be taken regularly for three to four weeks, though some as long as eight, before the full therapeutic effect occurs. Medication must then continue for at least four to nine months to prevent reoccurrence. Monitoring the discontinuation of anti-depressants is essential, due the risk of reoccurrence when abruptly stopped.

In 2006 the FDA approved the first transdermal (skin) patch, Emsam (selegiline), an MAOI inhibitor, for treatment of major depression. Using one low dose patch per day with none of the dietary restrictions associated with MAOI's should make life easier and less restrictive for patients.

Other, more radical treatment options are also available. Though these are undoubtedly out of the scope of FM, I include them for interest and completeness. Electroconvulsive therapy (ECT), once known as shock treatment, is used only for severe cases of depression which are not responsive to other treatments. Lower levels of shock are now administered than in previous times. Confusion and memory loss are possible side effects. Vagus nerve stimulation (VNS), in which a pacemaker-like device is implanted which sends electric impulses to the vargus nerve requires four or more medications to have been ineffective and the patient to be at least 18 years of age. Forty percent of patients have shown 50 percent or greater improvement. Side effects include hoarseness, sore throat, and shortness of breath. Transcranial magnetic stimulation (TMS), also known as repetitive transcranial magnetic stimulation (rTMS), was developed in 1985 and has been used in the treatment of mental illness since 1995. Electromagnets deliver short bursts of energy to stimulate nerve cells in the brain. The effect is comparable to a placebo and is used when the patient has not responded to traditional therapy.

Alternative medicines include St. John's wort, ephedra, gingko biloba, ☐chinacea, ginseng, and zinc, though no significant evidence has shown any of these to be beneficial. Care must be used when taking alternative medicines to consult a physician for potential drug interactions. Additionally, recent research has concluded that swimming with bottle nose dolphins for a period of at least two weeks may have some beneficial effect [9]. It could be assumed the benefit of this therapy may come more from doing something unusual, relaxing, and pleasurable than actually swimming with the dolphins. Perhaps snorkeling in the Caribbean or taking the long-dreamt-of pottery class may achieve similar results.

Obviously, for the FMer suffering from depression, the primary treatment is to control the fructose intake, thus allowing tryptophan to absorb. Psychotherapy and/or the support of other FMers may be needed to deal with the drastic change in life caused by FM.

Unfortunately, some will choose to self-medicate with drugs or alcohol. These simply exacerbate the depression through increased problems of physical, financial, legal, mental, and stress difficulties. It is debated whether substance abusers have an increased rate of depression…or if depression brings about substance abuse.

Though chemical imbalances in the brain are thought by many to be a cause of depression, these imbalances usually disappear upon completion of psychotherapy and this without medication. This suggests that perhaps the imbalance is a physical response to psychological distress. However the fact that some types of depression run in families (bi-polar and major depressive disorder), suggests that there is a biological connection. This can once again be debated by those arguing that social learning and coping factors learned within the family contribute to the hereditary link. My personal experience and opinion is that there is a chemical imbalance, which if severe enough, must be treated with medication aided by behavior and attitude modification.

One might wonder if the chemical imbalance is a result of other imbalances, such as those associated with FM as described at the beginning of this chapter.

Certain high blood pressure and arthritis medications can have a drug interaction which can bring about depression. Life events such as medical problems (like FM), financial difficulties, loss of loved ones, and loneliness experienced by those without proper coping skills are known triggers for depression. Elderly in institutions, diabetics, the socially isolated, and adolescents at the onset of puberty are at increased risk. People with other psychological disorders, especially anxiety disorders, have a higher rate of depression.

Commonly, those who suffer from depression share certain traits. They include pessimism, unrealistic expectations, overly self critical, low self-esteem, perfectionism, greater dependency needs, low self-efficacy (low self-worth), and external locus of control (getting one's sense of self from sources outside self, such as loved ones, need for recognition, and surroundings). For those who possess these traits or have a family history of depression, perhaps possible preemptive measures would aid in reducing depression occurrence. Counseling before depression or even classes or self-help books on building self-esteem may be beneficial.

Many of the traits mentioned above could be used to describe me. Thankfully, fewer apply today than in previous years. For example, if it were not for that trait of perfectionism, this book would have been published six months sooner.

After adolescence, women are twice as likely to suffer from depression as men. This holds true regardless of racial or ethnic background and is the same in eleven other countries as well. There have been many theories regarding the reasoning for this difference in rates. Among them are: hormonal differences, social role differences, and cultural differences. Many women experience pre-menstrual syndrome (PMS), with the emotional symptoms very closely mimicking depression. Additionally, post partum depression, which can, in extreme cases, lead to major depressive disorder, is thought to be due to the radical change in hormones experienced after birth. I experienced my first bout of major depressive disorder post partum. It is also interesting to note that one study has shown gender as a possible influence in FM, with women exhibiting more FM than men.[13]

Social role differences play an important part in the rate of depression differences by gender. While traditionally, men have had jobs and careers which allowed them to have defined schedules, time away from home, and fulfilling feedback, women have traditionally stayed at home. The homemaker's job, while important, can often be thankless, scheduleless or routine, and confining. All of these things can contribute to depression. Even today, when many women have satisfying careers outside the home, many still retain responsibility for housekeeping, child care, and meals, which can lead to feelings of being overwhelmed, a trigger for depression.

The rate difference between genders may be due to men being less likely to seek help. Additionally, men tend to self-medicate with alcohol or drugs more often, therefore the depression may simply be masked by substance abuse. This argument can be substantiated by looking at the Amish, where alcohol use is forbidden; in whom the depression rate for men and women is equal. Of course, culture differences can be closely associated with social differences. Additionally, with culture there is the question of reliability within the reported rates. It could be that in some cultures depression is simply under-reported due to cultural norms, allowances, and expectations.

This higher incidence of depression in women begins in adolescence. Until then, boys show an equal or even higher rate than girls. This leads us to realize other possible reasons for the higher rate in women are: hormonal, reproductive, genetic/biological factors, abuse and oppression, psychological and personality characteristics, different coping mechanisms, and social expectations. The reasons are unclear.

Victims' studies have shown an increased rate of depression among women who were: molested as children, raped as an adult, physically abused, mentally abused, or sexually harassed or abused. This may be due to these actions fostering low self esteem, feelings of helplessness, self-blame, and social isolation.

Seniors citizens also show a higher rate of depression in women than men. Attributing to this may be the reality that women statistically live longer, thus outliving their spouses and suffering the loss of a love one. This may also explain why unmarried or widowed seniors show a higher rate of depression. Other factors contributing to depression in senior citizen are: forced retirement, health problems, disability, age restrictions, caretaking responsibilities, lack of mobility, loss of driving privileges, and social isolation.

Children also suffer from depression. Faking illness, refusing to go to school, clinging to a parent, and worrying a parent may die, are indicators of depression in young children. For older children, sulking, negativity, feelings of being misunderstood, and grouchiness may be indicatory of depression. These symptoms make it difficult to diagnose depression in teens, since they are also associated with teen rebellion or emotional reactions to hormonal changes. However, they should not be overlooked since four out of one hundred teens are diagnosed as seriously depressed each year.

Whether income level plays a part is also subject to debate. Perhaps this income level factor has to do with the ability to get treatment, though studies have shown lower income sufferers are less likely to respond to treatment. Of course, higher incomes may allow people to participate in a greater variety of activities more often.

For those who have recovered from a bout with depression, the risk of recurrence increases with each successive depression. There are, however, steps one can take to increase feelings of self-worth and self-respect, which will aid in decreasing the risk of recurrence. I have survived two major bouts with depression and have adjusted my lifestyle and habits to include these recommendations, a few of which I have discovered myself and not seen listed in any other sources.

Ways to Battle Depression:

- Set a regular schedule, including a specific time for going to bed and getting up.
- Have a morning routine which includes dressing, shoes, hair, make-up or shaving.

- Maintain clean, orderly surroundings.
- Prioritize your life.
- Limit your responsibilities, feelings of being overwhelmed are a trigger.
- Maintain financial balance. Overwhelming debt is a loss of control.
- Keep goals attainable.
- Be social, especially when feelings say not to.
- Break large tasks into small ones which are not as overwhelming.
- Get plenty of regular exercise.
- Do not accept negative thinking.
- Keep active in hobbies and other enjoyable activities.
- Do not make major life decisions without consulting others when depressed.
- Set limits, such as not eating in front of the television.
- See a professional if needed.
- For the FMer taking control of your diet, as I have with organics, helps to achieve a feeling of control over food.

- Peer support can be invaluable in aiding self-acceptance and reducing the stigma attached to depression and seeking help. Sharing personal knowledge and coping strategies with others can help everyone involved as well as providing social support. By seeking peer support, one can obtain a feeling of greater control, which aids greatly in repressing depression. The fact that the support is coming from peers rather than being paternalistic (such as me sharing my experiences with my child) or hierarchical (such as in a patient/councilor situation) also contributes to success. Ultimately, the better one can feel about self and surroundings, the better they will do.

To help a depressed person:

- Be encouraging.
- Make the appointment for treatment, if necessary. You may also need to take the depressed person to the appointment.
- Assure that medications are being taken.

- Provide emotional support in the form of being understanding, patient, and affectionate.
- Listen to the sufferer.
- Do not disparage their thoughts and feelings, though gently pointing out realities and hopes can be of help.
- Invite them out; depressed people isolate themselves, so be insistent, yet respectful.
- Encourage activities; take a class with them.
- Encourage exercise; do it with them.
- Never accuse someone of faking depression, laziness, or not desiring to get better.
- Always report any talk of suicide.

Suicide is the third leading cause of death in the 15 to 24 age group. It must be taken seriously. Additionally, it is the eighth leading cause of death for men, and eleventh for people of all ages. Women attempt suicide three times as often as men. The key word there is "attempt," men succeed more often.

Why is the rate of suicide increasing? Many things may attribute to this increase: it is in the spotlight, creating more diagnosis; increased substance abuse; rising stress levels due to the changing job market and unemployment; an unhealthy focus on self; television, with its accompanying exposure to violence, lack of exercise, unrealistic lifestyles and images, and reduced social interaction; and a lack of commitment to a greater good.

Early screening and intervention helps prevent major depression with its potential for long term disability. Improving the ability of the primary care physician (PCP) to recognize depression, even mild cases, would aid in this effort. Additionally, PCP's increased understanding of the need to treat the disease through psychotherapy, rather than just the symptoms with medications, will aid in reducing depression rates.

As an FMer, if you seek help for depression, be sure your physician or therapist is aware of the FM and its accompanying tryptophan absorbency problems. You may wish to show him/her the first few pages of this chapter.

Reduced depression rates would also save expense in the form of reduced costs for employers though less absenteeism, turnover, and increased motivation as well as productivity. Nearly 19 million Americans suffer from depression resulting in direct and indirect costs of over $80 billion per year. As one of the leading causes of disability worldwide, depression demands research and respect as a disease.

Knowledge is power. Possessing this information may assist the FMer in battling this potentially disabling side effect of FM. Be aware of the symptoms. Take steps to minimize the grip or possibility of depression. Don't let FM or its partner, depression, win.

Bob's Point of View

My wife Debra was diagnosed with FM. The good news…we finally knew why she was always hurting. The bad news…life was about to become a little more complicated.

After searching the internet and printing food lists and any other information we could find, we realized that no two lists were the same. They were, in fact, quite contradictory. I then made a list of my own, including only foods which were okay on all the different lists. The resulting list was very small. As I sat and looked at it, I wondered what we would eat. "What kind of recipes could I make with that little list?" I thought. I wanted to cook a few things Deb could eat and see if she would start feeling better. There were only five veggies on the list, and one of them she didn't like.

I mean, come on….no canned corn, corn on the cob, corn tortillas, no tomatoes, tomato sauce, tomato paste, ketchup…no onions, garlic, carrots, peas. There goes Mexican, Italian, Chinese, stew, and my favorite, the hamburger corn casserole my mom made. I hate to talk about the negatives here, but that forbidden list was huge. I went through several cookbooks trying to alter some recipes without much luck. At least I had meat, potatoes, eggs, and dairy, which helped a little.

As the weeks passed, Debra became more and more frustrated. Breakfast was easy, but making lunch for herself, dinner for us, or shopping for tolerable foods was starting to get the best of her. I cooked when I could to take some of the burden off of her, but more than once, when I made the mistake of asking what she might want for dinner, she broke down in tears. This new lifestyle was overwhelming and she was tired of dealing with it. Shopping with her on weekends seemed to help. Reading labels while working our way down each isle showed the difficulty of finding anything without HFCS or other forbidden additives.

Keeping morale up was not easy, but I always tried to find the bright side somewhere. Then I began to get irritated myself. We did not have any good food around the house anymore and I could not even find a quick snack. Just as couples say "we're" pregnant...."we" have FM. Yes, Debra, the kids, and I were all in the same boat. Deb was the only one feeling the real pain, but we were all feeling the hunger.

As if the problems we were working through at home due to FM were not bad enough, try going to someone else's house for dinner. At first they would cook as they normally do. Deb would pick through trying to find something she could eat, not wanting to make a big deal of it. Then the questions would arise. "Can't you eat that?" "No." "Well, what can you eat?" Deb would then try to explain what she could not eat until I would interrupt and suggest she stick with what she could eat, it would not take as long. After explaining this, most people would just stare with a puzzled look on their faces. While the majority are still baffled, they will at least attempt to make a plan with Deb before cooking.

When we were first married, we learned that eating out, wine tasting, and trying different types of food was fun. We went to all the places in town (small town) and tried different things on the menu. This also gave us a good excuse to take a road trip by ourselves or with friends and family. Whenever we went on vacation, eating new and different food was beginning to take over as the best part of the trip.

This seems funny to me now, but when we first started going out after Deb was diagnosed with FM, no one was laughing. What was once a quiet, relaxing, romantic, fun night became a stressful, complicated evening without much romance or fun. We simply quit going out to dinner for a while. It just was not worth the money for the added stress it would bring.

Breakfast was still good. Thank goodness for breakfast! We could eat out while enjoying the restaurant and the atmosphere with few problems. Despite not being able to have syrup or jelly on her pancakes and steering clear of cured ham and sausage, breakfast was still a good time.

Lunch was a pain, but being cheaper than dinner we still went out occasionally. We would pick up our menus and study them, trying to discern something safe for Deb to eat. Usually before we had decided, an unsuspecting waitress would approach the table. "Run!" I thought, "You don't know what you're getting yourself into." No, this was not going to be an easy tip, with Deb asking if the gravy was made in house or came in a package. Does it have HFCS in it? MSG? Corn flour? Does the meat have a rub, brine, or a sauce on it? What are the veggies and can I substitute? By this time the confused looking server would usually force a smile and offer to ask the cook. Usually, she would return with "the cook's not sure," and offer an uneducated guess of her own.

By this time I would be a bit embarrassed. I understood Deb wanted to order something which would not make her spend the rest of the day in misery, but I'm just not the type to run the wait staff around in circles trying to accommodate me. If the food is not the best or the service is not good, rather than saying anything, I may not tip as well or simply not return, but normally, I am not one to complain.

Hopefully, by now we would find something easy, very basic, or (sigh) Deb might go on to the next choice on the menu and go through it all again. Yes, by this time I was irritated. We may have ended up having wonderful food, wine, or a good beer for me, but my patience and understanding were shot.

We had a few bad lunch experiences, but in the mean time we were learning. We were both new at this FM thing. We didn't know how to deal with it. We were in denial. We did not want to accept this new life. But we did learn patience. We gained experience and learned to have a good time. I guess you could say lunch was our practice, where we learned we could go out to dinner again and enjoy ourselves.

Admittedly, I miss the old days, when we could go out and eat or drink what ever we wanted to, but we've learned so much about food, additives, and preservatives, I am sure we eat healthier now. Though Deb still experiences pain, from unknowingly eating something bad or from just being defiant and eating a brownie, I encourage her that if she will eat cautiously for a few days in a row and get her system cleaned out, we can try something new in her diet.

We keep trying to add new foods to the okay list, or at least to the tolerable list.

The doctor says there are no long-term affects, but with the headaches, depression, bloating, and other symptoms we have associated with the way she eats, I think there is more to it than the doctors know at this time.

So what can I tell you, the reader? It will take time and patience. During that time, get on the internet and search for information which is increasing continually. Take control of your life, eat right, and exercise. This will all help with the associated depression. If someone you live with has FM, encourage them to eat foods they can easily tolerate for a few days then pick one of their favorite foods to try. If that food causes discomfort, depending on the severity, it may be able to be eaten in smaller quantities. Experimentation is the only way you can increase the size of the okay list. The best way to help you through this time is to help the FMer. There is a lot of good food out there, so look at it as a challenge. Life is still good!

The Rest of My Story

At the time of my diagnosis, my husband, Bob, and I had recently begun enjoying trying different wines and cheeses. After my diagnosis, that stopped. Wine is not my friend, especially the sweet wines I enjoy. I can, however, have very small amounts of very dry wine, though since I do not enjoy it, we mostly limit its use to cooking.

We also enjoyed trying new foods at new restaurants; since restaurants are now a dangerous source of frustration, this is no longer fun. I use the term dangerous because we never know for sure what is in the food. Also, the onions I had spent forty years learning to like, only to learn they are my enemy, are used universally in restaurants.

To say the depression which has been my nemesis for years has been defeated is premature. Unfortunately, the changes FM make, coupled with the frustration of the never-ending task of figuring out what to eat, exacerbated my depression. As I have learned more and feel more control over my food choices, I have continually improved in this area.

When I was first diagnosed, I would walk into the kitchen for meal preparation, realize I had no idea what I could eat or that I was weary of the few foods I knew were okay, and then walk out. I simply could not make a meal. Not eating was easier than trying to figure out what I could eat. Thankfully, Bob is better in the kitchen than I am anyway, so he took over completely. It took three months for me to attempt dinner. Time and confidence have given us the knowledge to prepare meals with little or no frustration. Dinner can, once again, be a delight.

The grocery store was another source of total despair. It was six months before I could shop by myself. What does one buy when their favorite section had previously been produce? This coupled with HFCS being listed on so many labels and I was lost. Try buying a loaf of bread without HFCS next time you go to the store. (Franz and Oro-Wheat now both make some) If you find hamburger buns without it, please let me know...since originally writing this, I found some! Oro-Wheat now offers hamburger buns without HFCS. They are expensive, but worth it. (This book has been two years in the making, so I had to make a few adjustments.) Organic buns can also be found in the organic food stores in larger cities. Of course, if you are extremely sensitive to fructans, these may not be an option. As always, read the label!

Unlike a weight-loss diet, cheating is no fun. Beyond the pain involved, I have noticed I get an FM "hangover." Systemic bloating is the most annoying price I pay. It is no fun feeling like a balloon. Add to this a headache, gas, lethargy, lack of sleep, and pain…well…cheating just is not worth it.

Extended family and friends are also affected by FM. They are afraid to make me sick. They are even more perplexed about what I can and cannot eat than I have been. My mom said one evening upon our arrival at her house, "I was going to have something ready to eat, but I just don't know what you can eat." As my daughters both have said, "Give me a list!" We can help alleviate some of the fear and frustration experienced by our friends and families by making and distributing lists of edibles and inedibles. Be sure to send periodic updates as your list grows.

Remaining cheerful and not whining can help them to know it is still okay for them to enjoy food and treats, regardless of how we eat.

Then there are those people, usually casual acquaintances or strangers, who react with disbelief when told about FM. It seems when people hear of a condition with which they are unfamiliar, from someone other than a physician, some have the tendency to disregard it as a fad or something made-up. I realize their opinion does not matter and will probably soon be changed as this condition becomes more well known.

I would love to say I have weathered all this very well, taken it in stride, so to speak, but I can not. I was, and sometimes, though rarely, still am a mess. Many tears have been shed. Early on, a television commercial which showed a juicy red apple reduced me to a sobbing mess. Forget the effect the actual produce department has produced. Incidentally, I am a chocoholic. But given a choice, I would easily give up chocolate before fruits and vegetables. Regrettably, both are in very short supply these days.

On the brighter side, today, more than two years after diagnosis, I'm doing much better. Physically and mentally I am in a much better place. Usually, I can view my eating restrictions as a challenge. Attitude, as in most things, is the majority of the battle. When I survive a difficult situation without getting depressed, angry or caving in, I can be proud of myself. When I do give in it is beginning to be a bit of a learning experience. I know I have no one to blame but myself. Often, I was the one who made the choice to eat whatever it was that made me sick. This helps me to think twice the next time before eating the forbidden fruit (or brownie).

If you have recently been diagnosed as an FMer, you may very well reach this point sooner than I did due to three reasons. First, there is more information available to help now. Upon diagnosis, my internet research revealed very little information or research. Just one year later, when researching the paper which was the basis for this book, there was, comparatively, a great deal of information. Of course, there is still much less than we would like to find. Also, my sincerest hope is for this book to encourage you in your acceptance and adjustment, as well as providing a resource for you, your family, and friends to understand your new life. Lastly, I was diagnosed about six weeks after my dad's death, about the same time the trauma of his death began to subside and reality hit. This resulted in two major losses and depression hitting on two fronts.

Ultimately, it is not just the restrictions which make life so difficult with FM, it is taking care, only to find myself in pain, bloated, and having no idea what I did wrong. Usually, it is those dastardly hidden onions I spent so many years learning to love which bring me to tears.

Appendix

Support Groups / Books

Support Groups

After a great deal of searching, below are the on-line support groups I have found which discuss FM. Obviously, I am more familiar with some than with others. The leg work has been done for you, so you decide which will work for you.

* One of the best support sites I have found is an easy name to remember, for good reason. With a current membership of 78, it is not unusual to find at least a few fellow members on at the same time. The site reports there were recently 28 members online simultaneously. Ease of use, coupled with various topic headings, make this a very user-friendly site. http://fructosesucks.com/

* The following support group is an Australian support group which closely adheres to Dr. Sue Shepperd's Low Fodmap ™ diet. It has a large membership (304 as of this writing) and was started in

December 2006. While it can provide a great deal of support with frequent postings, I find it rather tedious at times to follow. Additionally, Dr. Shepperd focuses on gluten/wheat free, which is not my primary problem. She also says I should be able to have things like tomato base pasta sauces, soda pop, and Splenda sweetener, which I clearly cannot have.

http://health.groups.yahoo.com/group/fructose_malab sorption_australia

* This support group is new (February 09) with only 18 members as of this writing. The few postings so far show it may end up being a good support system.

http://health.groups.yahoo.com/group/fructose_malab sorption/

* This is a portion of A.V Thompson's (British Columbia, Canada), weblog. Ms. Thompson has an amazing aptitude for putting a humorous slant on this oh-so-frustrating condition. Whether you ever post or not, I highly recommend this site for a welcome laugh.

http://avthompson.wordpress.com/what-is-fructose-malabsorption-disorder/

* For those with children with FM, this blog site may be especially helpful. I also found it to be quite interesting.
http://fructosemalabsorptioninchildren.blogspot.com/

* I found a bit of discussion regarding FM on this recipe site. Perhaps with a bit of search, we can find some more recipes!
http://www.recipezaar.com/bb/viewtopic.zsp?p=4510349#4510349

* If you have a baby who is has FM, you may be able to find some of the specialized support which this would require on this site.
http://www.infantrefluxdisease.com

* Another site companionship for those with a child with FM may be this blog.
http://fructosemalabsorptioninchildren.blogspot.com/2008/11/toddler-night-waking-when-will-it-stop.html

137

*   This is a site for parents of kids with allergies. There are some postings regarding FM on it. http://www.kidswithfoodallergies.org/resourcesnew.php

*   Another site for parents of children with FM could commiserate with other parents of children with a variety of health problems is http://www.askmoxie.org/2008/08/message-boards-for-kids-medical-issues.html

*   Though at first glance this seems to be a site dedicated to HFI, further digging shows there are many confused FMer's as well as a few with a handle on the FM thing on this site. http://www.dailystrength.org/c/Fructose_Intolerance/forum/5523524-intolerance-vs-malabsorption

*   You can find some discussion of FM on this site. http://www.ibsgroup.org/forums/index.php?showtopic=99573

*   Some, especially those who are extremely sensitive to wheat, may find this site helpful.
http://forums.glutenfree.com/post61509.html

Books

Living with Dietary Fructose Intolerance

A Guide to Managing Your Life
With This New Diagnosis

By: Judy Smith,
A Fellow DFI Patient

Up until now, Judy Smith has had the only book I have been able to locate on the subject of FM (though she does use an older term for it) and the only one I have heard mentioned on any of the support sites. She includes her experiences, suggestions, and 26 recipes. I found it to be somewhat encouraging early on, as well as a quick read

.

Low Fodmap™ Diet
Fructose Malabsorption
Food Shopping Guide
4th Edition

By: Dr. Sue Shepherd

Dr. Shepherd, a practicing dietitian in Australia, is one of the most well-known authorities on the subject of FM. This book includes a short introduction, then lists of acceptable foods by class, including color pictures of brand packaging. I am not sure if some of the discrepancies between her lists in the book and what can actually be eaten stem from her being in Australia. For instance, she lists Coca Cola as okay because most other countries make it with cane sugar, though in the United States it clearly contains HFCS. Also, she lists tomato saucy items as okay.

Dr. Shepherd has also written three books for those with FM:
"Irresistible for the Irritable"
"Two Irresistible for the Irritable"
"Gluten Free Cooking"

We have not yet ordered any of these award-winning and best-selling books. We hoped to first come up with recipes on our own for inclusion in this book.

Bob's List

This is the list Bob compiled of foods which are on all six lists as acceptable foods.

Protein	Veggies	Dairy	Breads& Cereals	Carbs
Beef	Asparagus #	Milk	Ezekiel Bread	
				Potatoes
Pork	Peppers *	Cheese	Sprouted Grain Bread	
				Pasta
Chicken	Cauliflower *	Butter	Unsweet-ened bread	
Turkey	Celery	Sour Cream	Oatmeal	
Venison	Spinach	Unsweetened Yogurt	White Rice	
Fish	Mushrooms			
Nuts*				
Tofu				
Eggs				
Seafood				

* May cause gas – some people report problems with nuts

Fructans, since then we have found it on most "no" lists, though I can eat it without problems

While not on the original list, we have added mushrooms and nuts to this list.

Can Eat

Remember, when using this or any list in this book, individual tolerances vary. The list below is only a starting point. Be sure to read the ingredients. Feel free to copy this list for your own use.

Food		Fructose	Glucose
Alcohol			
	Gin		
	Rum		
	Vodka		
	Saki		
	Tequila-despite being made from agave, I seem to tolerate small amounts		
	Wine - Dry Only		
	Whiskey		
Bananas		2.7	4.2
Bean Sprouts	good sub for onions		
Beans - Dried Legumes			
Beef			
Berries	(black, blue, raspberries, etc.)		
Black-eyed Peas		0.2	0.2
Buckwheat			

Buckwheat Pancakes			
Food		**Fructose**	**Glucose**
Butter	Real butter only		
Buttermilk			
Cauliflower		0.8	0.9
Cabbage			
	Chinese	0.6	0.8
	Green	1.5	1.7
	Red	1.5	1.7
Cassava Root		0.1	0.1
Celery	Though the US Dept of Agriculture source lists celery as having a small amount of polyols in the form of mannitol, I can find no other source which agrees with this. I have had no problems with celery.	0.5	0.4
Cereal	limited types- organic without wheat, corn, molasses, or honey is best		
Cheese			
	American - pasteurized processed	0	0.1
	Cheddar	0	0.1
	Cream	0	0
	Mozzarella	0	0
	Ricotta	0	0
Chicken			
Chicory Roots		0.1	0.1

Chives		0.3	0.4
Coffee			
Collard Greens			
Cottage Cheese		0	0
Cranberries			
Cranberry Juice	Be careful of sweetener		
Dandelion Greens		0.4	0.5
Eggplant - raw		1.5	1.6
Eggs			
Fish			
Flour Tortilla	Depending on your ability to handle flour		
Graham Crackers	Read Ingredients		
Grapefruit		1.2	1.3
Jackfruit		1.4	1.4
Kale		0.2	0.3
Kiwi	Note: US Dept. of Agriculture lists as 4.4/5, NutritionData.com lists as 4.4/4.1, personally, I can not eat them	4.4	5
Kohlrabi		1.2	1.3
Lamb			
Lays Potato Chips	Check ingredients, last bag I had included corn oil, it was not pretty!		

Lemons		0.9	1.0
Lettuce			
	Cos	0.8	0.4
	Romaine	0.8	0.4
Limes		0.2	0.2
Milk			
Mushrooms	Thankfully!	0.2	1.5
Mustard Greens		0.3	0.4
Nuts	Almonds	0.9	1.2
	Cashews	0.8	0.8
	Filberts (Hazelnuts)	0.7	0.7
	Macadamia	0.7	0.7
	Peanuts		
	Pecans	0.4	0.4
	Pine Nuts	0.7	0.7
	Pistachio	1.3	2.3
	Walnuts, black	0.5	0.5
Oatmeal			
Olives	Supposed to...I hate them		
Orange			
Passion Fruit		3.1	4.0
Pasta			
Peanut Butter			
Peanuts		0	0.2
Peppers, sweet	Green only	1.12	1.16
Pinto Beans		0	0
Pistachios		0.1	0.2
Pomegranates		4.7	5.0
Pork			
Potatoes			

	Red	0.3	0.4
	Russet	0.32	0.37
	White	0.3	0.5
Raspberries		3.9	4.3
Rhubarb		0.4	0.4
Rutabaga		1.4	3.2
Rice			
	White		0.2
	Wild	0.9	0.9
Squash,	summer, all varieties	0.9	0.7
Squash, winter			
	Butternut	1.0	1.0
	Pumpkin	1.4	1.7
Seafood			
Sesame Flour		1.9	2.4
Snap peas			
Sour Cream			
Soy Milk			
Soy Sauce	some report problems		
Spices			
	Basil-Dried	7.5	7.5
	Basil-Fresh	0.2	0.2
	Cloves	10.7	11.4
	Curry Powder	7.9	11.4
	Oregano	1.1	1.9
	Mustard Seed	0.2	28.8
	Parsley	4.2	27.6
	Poppy Seed	2.9	3.7
Spinach		0.1	0.1
Sweet Potato		0.7	1.0
Swiss Chard		0.2	0.4
Tea	With allowed		

	sweeteners only		
Tofu			
Tortellini	Check the ingredients		
Triscuits			
Turkey			
Turnip Greens		0.3	0.5
Unsweetened Yogurt			
Venison			
Vinegar			
	Balsamic	7.3	7.5
	White, Distilled		
Watercress		0.1	0.4
Wax gourd		0.5	0.5
Yogurt, plain	Read ingredients! Most contain HFCS, honey, or molasses	0	3.2
Zucchini			

Notes:

Lemon juice: (squeeze bottle) there is an amazing difference between organic and non-organic. We were astounded at the difference. The organic is so far superior we now cringe if we are unable to find it.

Can Not Eat

Remember, when using this or any list in this book, individual tolerances vary. The list below is only a starting point. Be sure to read the ingredients. Feel free to copy this list for your own use.

Food		Fructose	Glucose	Polyols
Alfalfa Sprouts		0.2	0.1	
Apples		5.9	2.4	
Apricots		1.2	3.3	*
Agave		42.8	3.5	
Bacon	Processed with honey, brown sugar, or other unacceptable sugars			
Beans, green		1.2	0.9	
Beer				
	Light	0	0.6	*
	Regular	0.2	1.0	*
	Cooler	3.9	3.0	
Beet Green				
Blackberries		2.4	2.3	
Blueberries		5.0	4.9	

Brandy, cherry		16.1	16.5	*
Breath Freshening Candies				*
	Polyols in the form of mannitol-that's what gives them their cooling, fresh feel			
Broad beans		0.9	0.4	
Brussels Sprouts		0.9	0.8	
Carambola		3.2	3.1	
Carrots		0.55	0.59	*
Carrots, baby		1.0	1.04	*
Cherries, sweet		5.4	6.6	*
Cherries, sour		3.5	4.2	*
Chewing Gum				*
Chickpeas		0.3	0.2	
Chocolate				*
Chocolate Milk				*
Coconut				
Corn		0.48	0.5	
Cucumbers		0.9	0.8	*
Currents		3.5	3.2	
Dates - medjool		31.9	33.7	*
Dates - deglet noor		19.6	19.9	*
Eggplant - fried		1.9	1.7	

Figs		2.8	3.7	
Fruit-juice				
Grapes		8.1	7.2	
Green Onions				
Guacamole				
Guava		1.9	1.2	
High-Fructose Corn Syrup		varies - see chapter on HFCS		
Honey		40.9	35.7	
Jerusalem Artichoke		0.8	0.6	
Kiwi		4.4	4.1	
Leeks		1.5	1.1	
Lettuce				
	Boston	0.5	0.4	
	Bib	0.5	0.4	
	Cos	0.8	0.4	
	Green leaf	0.43	0.36	
	Iceberg	1.0	0.9	
	Romaine	0.8	0.4	
Lemon juice	I can have this	1.1	1.0	
Lentil Beans		0.3	0.1	
Mandarin Oranges aka: tangerines		2.4	2.1	
Mangos		2.9	0.7	
Meats which are cured such as bacon, sausage, lunchmeats				
Meats which are breaded (unless you know what the breading is)				
Melon				

	Cantaloupe	1.8	1.2	
	Honeydew	3.0	2.7	
	Watermelon	3.4	1.6	
Mint				
Molasses		12.8	11.9	
Ming Beans		0.6	0.4	
Nectarines		1.1	1.2	*
Nuts				
	Walnuts, English	0.9	0.8	
Okra		1.0	0.8	
Onions		1.3	2.0	*
	Sweet	2.0	2.2	*
Oranges	This disagrees with the information I have found elsewhere. I can eat small ones	2.3	2.0	
Papaya		2.7	1.4	
Peaches		1.3	1.1	*
Pears		6.4	1.9	*
Peas		0.4	0.1	
Peppers, sweet, red		2.3	1.9	
Persimmons		5.6	5.4	
Pickles				
	Dill or Kosher	0.4	0.9	
	Sweet (including breading & butter)	8.8	9.2	
Pineapple		2.1	2.9	
Plums		3.1	5.1	
Prunes		14.8	28.7	*
Radishes		0.7	1.1	*
Raisins		29.7	27.8	
Salsify, black		0.1	0	
Scallions				
Shallots		0.3	0.4	*

Sausage				
Soda Pop	**Not if there is HFCS or inverted sugar**			
	Cola	4.4	4.0	
	Diet - Artificial Sweeteners	0	0	
	Ginger Ale	3.7	3.1	
	Lemon-lime	6.1	4.1	
	Root Beer	3.2	3.2	
Soy Beans		0.5	0.2	
	cooked	0.2	0.1	
Spices				
	Chili Powder	42.9	21.4	
	Cinnamon, ground	11.1	10.4	
	Ginger	17.8	12.2	
	Paprika	67.11	26.3	
	Turmeric	4.5	3.8	
Star fruit				
Strawberries		2.4	1.9	
Tangerines (mandarin oranges)		2.4	2.1	
Tomotillos				
Tomatoes		1.4	1.3	
Vinegar				
	Cider	3	1	
Wheat		0.2	0.2	*
Wine - Sweet				

Many condiments (tomato sauce, barbecue sauce, relish, sweet and sour sauce, and plum sauce)

Chai tea at coffee places

Notes:

Toothpaste: Be careful, most toothpastes are sweetened with "bad" sweeteners…as always, check the ingredients. Check the natural food store for organic toothpastes. But, as always, these may contain ingredients which of off limits also, so…read ingredients.

Maybe

Remember, when using this or any list in this book, individual tolerances vary. The list below is only a starting point. Be sure to read the ingredients. Feel free to copy this list for your own use.

Food		Fructose	Glucose
Amaranth, whole grain		0.1	0.4
Artichokes		0.6	1.5
Asparagus		1.0	0.7
Avocado		0.2	0.5
Bananas			
Beets		0.2	0.2
Berries - Most			
Broccoli		0.7	0.4
Carrots		1	1
Corn Tortillas		0	0.1
Citrus fruits			
Coconut			
	Raw	1.4	2.0
	Dried, flaked	0.2	0.6
Cucumbers		0.9	1
Cumquats			
Green Onion Tops (green part)			
Kiwi			
Lima Beans		0.6	
Orange			
Passion fruit			
Rye Flour		0.3	0.5
Squash			

Sweet potatoes		
Sunflower seeds		
Yams		
Yogurt	read it!	
Ham		
Wheat bread		
Wheat cereal		
Wheat pasta		
Wheat crackers		

Avoid or limit some foods that contain wheat, though it is not necessary to avoid all foods containing wheat as strictly as a diet for celiac disease (condiments, soups, etc). Different people have different tolerances for wheat. Avoid or limit the following:

Snacks

Remember, when using this or any list in this book, individual tolerances vary. The list below is only a starting point. Feel free to copy this list for your own use.

Item	Notes	Limited Quantity	Maybe
Bagel	be careful of ingredients, most have HFCS	X	
Bagel w/cream cheese			
Bagel w/cream cheese & jelly	be sure the jelly is one you can eat	X	
Banana		X	
Broccoli		X	
Cauliflower		X	
Celery Stick			
Celery with Cream Cheese			
Celery with Peanut Butter	PB varies, most contain HFCS, read labels		
Cheese			
Cheeze-its	original	X	X
Dried Bananas	be careful of ingredients - some sweeten with honey	X	X
Dried Cranberries	be careful of ingredients - some contain HFCS-read	X	X

	ingredients		
Egg - Boiled			
Glee Gum	Available at natural food stores or http://www.gleegum.com		X
Ice Cream	Certain kinds only-read ingredients	X	X
Jerky – rarely	be careful of ingredients – almost all contain bad stuff		
Lay's Potato Chips	Original only		
Nuts	check the fructose: glucose ratio list for kinds	X	
Orange Sections		X	
Pita Chips	watch ingredients		
Pringles Original	watch ingredients	X	X
Lundberg Rice Chips	www.lundberg.com		
RJ's Natural Soft-Eating Licorice- raspberry only	Also available on Amazon.com The black is unacceptable, it contains molasses. http://www.rjslicorice.co.nz/RJs_Natural_Soft_Eating_Range_16.aspx	X	
Rye Crackers	watch ingredients- Finn Crisps have only rye, yeast, and salt --- I have not tried these, I do not care for rye		
Smoked Salmon			
Soda Crackers	be careful of ingredients, most have HFCS		

String Cheese			
Sugar Snap Peas		X	
Triscuits	original, avoid if you are wheat sensitive	X	
Yogurt	organic, plain & vanilla...most others have HFCS		
Zucchini Slices		X	

Notes:

Gum: Be careful of gum, almost all gums are sweetened with sorbitol. Though not high on flavor, Glee gum is sweetened with cane sugar so it may not be as good for your teeth, but at least you can chew gum occasionally.

Chips: Remember corn can be problematic, so chips which include corn are not recommended. "Natural" potato chips may be less likely to contain bad ingredients, though label reading is still essential due to added things like onion powder and garlic. Be aware of the kind of potato used in the chips.

Soda: Check the natural food store for root beer or cream soda. I found Cascade Root Beer, brewed in Portland, Oregon. Remember, quantity is key to drinking soda.

Sugars & Sweeteners List

Repeated from the Sugars & Sweeteners Chapter

Remember, when using this or any list in this book, individual tolerances vary. The list below is only a starting point. Feel free to copy this list for your own use.

The following chart is an adaptation of the "Sugars & Sweeteners" chart on the Boston University website for hereditary fructose intolerance (HFI) [11]. (Used by permission.) The original chart includes a wide variety of sugars and sweeteners which are not common and for those of us hoping to simplify and understand, can be rather overwhelming so we have provided this condensed version listing the more common sweeteners. Additionally, since the original chart was designed for HFI patients (thus resulting in more confusion for the FMer), we have revised it somewhat for the FMer. The tolerance column has been changed to reflect the FMer's tolerance as gleaned from my experience coupled with comments from other FMer's on the internet. Remember, tolerance levels may differ and quantity is a factor. Determine your own tolerance levels. The "?" in the tolerance column is an indication that tolerance seems to vary widely.

Sugar Sweetener	Description	Tolerance
Agave Syrup	From the blue agave cactus. Commonly used in Tex-Mex foods, tequila, margaritas, soft drinks. High in fructose.	No

Sugar Sweetener	Description	Tolerance
Aspartame	Sugar substitute known as Equal, NutraSweet, NutraTase. FDA approved. Scientifically studied in depth. Some may be sensitive to headaches. Derived from amino acids.	No
Barley Malt Syrup	From sprouted grains of barley, kiln dried and cooked with water.	?
Beet Sugar	Sucrose. Same structure as cane sugar, but may produce different product results because of .05 differences in minerals and proteins. More common in Europe than the U.S	No
Brown Rice Syrup	Made from brown rice. High protein content. Likely contains sucrose.	?
Brown Sugar	Sucrose coated with molasses.	No
Cane Sugar	Sucrose. Table sugar.	Yes

Sugar Sweetener	Description	Tolerance
Corn Starch	Derived from corn. Composed of straight or branched chains of glucose.	No
Corn Sugar	Produced from corn starch. Contains glucose and maltose molecules.	No
Corn Syrup	Glucose and water. Usually produced from cornstarch. The problem is that in making the syrup, it may have either maltose and/or fructose added.	No
Corn Syrup Solids	Dried glucose syrup.	No
Confectioners Sugar	Sucrose. A chemical combination of glucose and fructose.	Yes
Date Sugar	Made from dried, pulverized dates. Likely contains sucrose.	No

Sugar Sweetener	Description	Tolerance
Dextrin	Glucose molecules linked together in chains. Does not break down to pure dextrose.	Yes
Dextrose	Single glucose molecule. Simple sugar.	Yes
Evaporated Cane Sugar	Sucrose. Another name for sugar cane juice.	Yes
Fructose	Simple sugar of fructose molecules. Sometimes called fruit sugar. Made of 6 carbons.	No
Fruit Juice Sweeteners	Derived from grapes, apples or pears, heated to reduce water leaving a sweeter more concentrated juice. Almost pure fructose.	No
Glucose	Simple sugar. The chemical sugar structure of blood sugar. Made of 6 carbons.	Yes

Sugar Sweetener	Description	Tolerance
Granulated sugar	Table sugar. Sucrose. Can be tolerated only if it is pure cane sugar, not beet sugar.	?
High Fructose Corn Syrup (HFCS)	Enzymetically converted from corn syrup to contain 42% - 90% fructose. Raises triglyceride levels and may increase risk of heart disease. See the chapter on HFCS.	No
Honey	Natural syrup containing about 35% glucose, 40% fructose, 25 % water	No
Inverted Sugar	Created by combining sugar syrup with cream of tarter or lemon juice and heating, breaking sucrose down to components glucose and fructose.	No
Isoglucose	Another name for High Fructose Corn Syrup (HFCS).	No

Sugar Sweetener	Description	Tolerance
Isomalt	Polyol	No
Levulose	Contains fructose.	No
Maltitol	Sugar alcohol form of maltose (glucose). This is a polyol.	No
Maltose	Linked glucose molecules that rapidly break down to glucose in the intestine.	Yes
Maple Syrup	Mostly sucrose. Contains some invert sugar.	No
Molasses	By-product of sugar cane with 24% water. Fructose level varies. Three kinds. Light (sweetest), Medium (darker and less sweet), Blackstrap (very dark, slightly sweet with distinctive flavor. Good source of calcium and iron)	No

Sugar Sweetener	Description	Tolerance
Molasses Sugar	Dark muscovado sugar with extra molasses.	No
Raffinose	A trisaccharide found in grains, legumes and some vegetables. Gas forming.	?
Raw Sugar	Sucrose. Equal parts glucose and fructose, a chemical combination of glucose and fructose.	Yes
Saccharin	Sugar substitute. Not as commonly used as in the past. Known as Sweet N' Low, Sugar Twin, Sucryl, Featherweight. FDA approved. More than 6 servings per day may increase bladder cancer risk. (No longer approved for use in Canada)	No
Sorbitol	Sugar alcohol. Common in fruits, particularly skin of ripe berries, cherries and plums. Used in sugar free foods. Causes diarrhea. Converted back to fructose. This is a polyol.	No
Splenda	A sugar substitute. This is a chemically modified sucrose molecule that □china be digested.	No

Sugar Sweetener	Description	Tolerance
Stevia	Natural sweetener from a South American plant. 30 % sweeter than sugar. Used extensively in Japan, China, Korea, Israel, Brazil and Paraguay with no side effects reported. Known as Stevioside. Has not been rigorously tested for safety. No consistent manufacturing regulations.	Yes
Sucralose	Chemical name for Splenda, a sugar substitute. Large molecule not digested.	No
Sucrose	Naturally occurring sugar made from sugar cane or sugar beets. Commonly referred to as sugar and table sugar. Chemical combination of glucose and fructose. Tolerated if from cane but not from beets.	?
Sucrose Syrups	Also known as Refiner's syrup. By product of sugar refining. 18% water, 1 part sucrose to two parts invert sugar.	No
Sugar	Common name for sucrose, a chemical combination of glucose and fructose.	Yes

Sugar Sweetener	Description	Tolerance
Xylitol	Sugar alcohol. Obtained from fruits and berries. Also from birch trees and known as birch sugar. May causes diarrhea.	?

Fructans

For more information on fructans, in easy to understand English, check the following website. I found this at the last minute before publication. I avoided incorporating any of it into this book because I wanted it all, which would have violated the author. http://www.raisin-hell.com/2008/11/fructans-inulin.html

Please note: This list is not necessarily all-inclusive. We have included all that we have been able to find.

Artichoke

Asparagus

Barley (very young)

Chives

Garlic

Leek

Onion

Rye

Wheat

A couple of sources I have found include banana.

Vitamin D List

Remember, when using this or any list in this book, individual tolerances vary. The list below is only a starting point. Feel free to copy this list for your own use.

Foods High in Vitamin D

USDS Recommended Daily Amount = 400IU

Food		IU*
Beef Kidneys		32
Beef Liver		16
Butter		56
Caviar		232
Cheese		
	Cheddar	12
	Parmesan	28
	Swiss	44
Clams		4
Cream - heavy whipping		52
Egg		35
Egg Yoke		107
Milk		
	Evaporated, canned	80
	Whole	40
	2%	43
	1%	52
	Non-fat	41
	Goat	12
	Human	4

Mushrooms - white		181
Mushrooms - canned		21
Mushrooms - cooked		21
Soymilk		49
Fish		
	Catfish	500
	Cod	44
	Flounder	60
	Halibut	600
	Herring	1628
	Mackerel	360
	Sole	60
Oysters		320
Shrimp		152

Tryptophan List

Remember, when using this or any list in this book, individual tolerances vary. The list below is only a starting point. Feel free to copy this list for your own use.

Foods High in Tryptophan

Bananas
Chicken
Cod
Halibut
Lamb
Milk
Mustard Greens
Salmon
Sesame Seed
Shrimp
Snapper
Soybeans
Spinach
Tuna
Turkey

A far more extensive and detailed list may be found at http://whfoods.org/genpage.php?tname=nutrient&dbid=103#foodsources

Newbie List

If you have just been diagnosed with FM, you will need to "cleanse." Start with Bob's List and create what you can for meals. Realizing this can be very difficult and rather monotonous, we have provided a list of possible meal items. As always, be sure to check labels before using an ingredient.

After you are "clean" for a while, you can begin adding, one at a time, other foods.

Breakfast
Eggs
>
> soft boiled
> hard boiled
> fried
> scrambled
> poached

Omelet
Oatmeal
Creamed Eggs
Uncle Sam Cereal
Rice
Camp Breakfast
Uncured Bacon
Hash browns
Fried Potatoes

Snacks
Celery Sticks
Boiled Egg
Nuts
Celery stuffed with
Cream Cheese
String Cheese

Cheese
Spoon of Peanut
Butter

Lunch

Turkey Pieces
1/2 Grilled Cheese Sandwich (with
acceptable bread)
Leftovers from Dinner
Lettuce Wraps
1/2 Meat or Fish Sandwich (with
acceptable bread)
Tuna Salad
Egg Salad

Dinner

Main Course

Lemon Chicken
Fried Chicken
Pork Chops
Burger Gravy
Kabobs
Stuffed Potato
Ground Meat Patties topped w/cheese (cream cheese
works well for this)
Grilled Fish
Quiche-without crust or with shredded
potato crust

Carbs

Pesto Pasta
Baked Potato
Fried Potato
Mashed Potato

Veggies

Get creative with your vegetable course. Steam, grill, stir-
fry, dry-fry, and mix and match

173

- Broccoli
- Cauliflower
- Zucchini
- Asparagus
- Mushrooms

Back to Basics List

If you are stressed about what to make for a meal, just go back to basics. Pick an item from each column, and voila' you have a balanced meal. You can skip the fats column; most of us get enough fat without purposely planning for it. If any of these bother you, cross it out. If you find others, add to the list.

Protein	Fruit & Vegetable	Carbo-hydrate	Dairy	Fat
Beef	Banana	Black-Eyed Peas	Buttermilk	Butter
Black Beans	Bean Sprouts	Cereal	Cheese	Olive Oil
Buffalo	Berries	Oatmeal	Ice Cream	Canola Oil
Chicken	Cauliflower	Pasta	Milk	
Eggs	Cabbage	Potatoes	Yogurt	
Fish	Casaba Root	Rice		
Lamb	Celery	Sweet Potato		
Navy Beans	Chicory Root			
Nuts	Collard Greens			
Peanut Butter	Dandelion Greens			
Pintos Beans	Eggplant			

Protein	Fruit & Vegetable	Carbo-hydrate	Dairy	Fat
Pork	Grapefruit			
Seafood	Green Peppers			
Tofu	Jackfruit			
Turkey	Kale			
Venison	Kiwi			
	Kohlrabi			
	Lettuce			
	Mushroom			
	Mustard Greens			
	Olives			
	Orange			
	Passion Fruit			
	Pome-granates			
	Raspberry			
	Rhubarb			
	Rutabaga			
	Squash			
	Snap Peas			
	Spinach			
	Swiss Chard			
	Turnip Greens			
	Watercress			
	Zucchini			

THE HEALTHY EATING PYRAMID

Department of Nutrition, Harvard School of Public Health

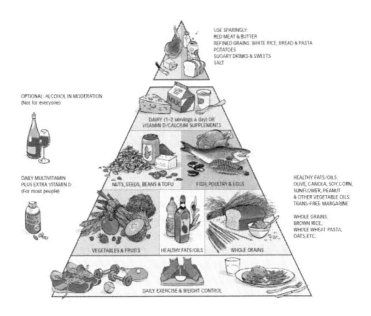

For more information about the Healthy Eating Pyramid:

WWW.THE NUTRITION SOURCE.ORG

Eat, Drink, and Be Healthy
by Walter C. Willett, M.D. and Patrick J. Skerrett (2005)
Free Press/Simon & Schuster Inc.

Copyright © 2008. For more information about The Healthy Eating Pyramid, please see The Nutrition Source, Department of Nutrition, Harvard School of Public Health, http://www.thenutritionsource.org, and Eat, Drink, and Be Healthy, by Walter C. Willett, M.D. and Patrick J. Skerrett (2005), Free Press/Simon & Schuster Inc.
Used by permission

Recipes

This is the chapter for which you have been waiting. Or, perhaps you've done what we would, perused the table of contents, then skipped right to the meat and potatoes, otherwise known as recipes.

Before you jump into cooking, or at least thinking about it, how about a few healthy food basics? Protein, fruits, vegetables, carbohydrates, dairy, and fats are the basics of any good diet. You are no doubt familiar with the food pyramid. For meal preparation, you now know all you really need to know.

Okay, maybe it is not quite that simple, but it can be close. Simply take a look at the list on page 171, choose one food from each category, and you have a meal. Stress is overrated. So if you are at a loss for what to make for dinner, just go back to basics. Meals do not need to be fancy, complicated, or involved. If you are still having problems, see the Newbie List.

During these days of instant and fast food, for those who are a bit rusty on the basics, an excellent resource may be found on the Harvard School of

Public Health website at

http://www.hsph.harvard.edu/nutritionsource/what-should-you-eat/pyramid/.

Amazing Spaghetti Sauce

2 lb. ground turkey
1 stick butter
1 bunch asparagus – ½ the tops minced, the rest diced
    (or broccoli if you can't tolerate asparagus)
½ stalk celery – finely minced
1 stalk celery - diced
1 – 2 cups mushrooms – chopped or 3 cans
1 pint heavy cream (aka whipping cream)
1 pint half and half
3 Tablespoons flour
Salt & Pepper to taste
Juice from mushrooms
If you can tolerate green onions, they are great in this.

Brown ground turkey in large skillet.

While turkey is browning, heat heavy cream and half and half in separate saucepan. Do not boil.

Just before turkey is done, add the butter, asparagus, celery, and mushrooms. When turkey is done, turn the heat down, add flour and mix well.

Add the milk mixture and juice from the mushrooms. Simmer.

Burger Gravy

1 Pound Ground Meat
      (We use beef, turkey, or buffalo. It is not as
flavorful with turkey.)
Flour
Milk
Salt
Pepper

Brown the meat in a skillet on medium high heat.
Add flour until it stays white and will not absorb
anymore. Due to the difference in amounts of fat in
ground meat it is difficult to give an amount. Add
about two cups of milk. If the gravy begins to thicken
too much, add more milk. Simmer at a slight boil for
a few minutes then reduce to low or medium low.
The longer you heat (up to an hour), the better the
flavor. Salt and pepper to taste.

Spoon over either mashed or baked (cut in pieces)
potatoes or noodles.

I usually use baked potatoes because they are quick
and easy in the microwave. This is a very easy dish to
throw together.

Camp Breakfast # 1

4-5 Medium Potatoes
½ pound Ground Meat, cooked
6 slices uncured bacon, cooked and cut or crumbled
4 Eggs
1-2 Cups Cheese
1 Cup Veggies of Choice, sliced or cubed
½ cup chopped bell peppers
Salt
Pepper

Fry potatoes, adding vegetables and cooked meat just before done. Turn the heat down to low. Add the eggs and fold in about three times only. Top with cheese and cover. When cheese has melted, remove from burner and serve.

If you stir your eggs in too long the dish will become dry. The eggs will cook as the cheese melts.

Good topped with sour cream and for other family members, salsa (but not for the FMer!)

Works well wrapped in a tortilla as a breakfast burrito.

Nice meal for cleaning out your refrigerator.

Camp Breakfast #2
Simpler version

Cooked hash browns or fried potatoes
Cooked ground meat
Chopped veggies of your choice
Cheese (grated)
4-6 Eggs (very lightly mixed)
Salt
Pepper

Place a layer of potatoes on the bottom of a baking dish. Top this with a layer of ground meat. Follow this with a layer of veggies. Top with the grated cheese. Pour the eggs over the whole thing. Salt and pepper to taste. Cover with foil and bake in a 350° oven for 15-20 minutes. Take the foil off the last 5 minutes.

Cheese Pie

1 - 9 Inch Graham Cracker Crust (optional)
1 - 8 Ounce Package Cream Cheese, Softened
1 – 14 Ounce Can Sweetened Condensed Milk
    (Check the ingredients)
1/3 Cup Lemon Juice
1 teaspoon Vanilla

Beat the cream cheese until light and fluffy. Add the sweetened condensed milk and blend thoroughly. Stir in lemon juice and vanilla. Pour into crust, if using, or dessert cups. Chill at least three hours. The flavor improves if it can be chilled 24 hours.

A few ripe raspberries or blackberries squashed and allowed to "juice" while the pie is chilling would make a wonderful topping.

Remember: If you can eat this, consume only very small quantities. It is very high in sugar.

Chinese Burger Helper

2 Cups Warm Water
1 ½ -2 Pounds Ground Meat
½ teaspoon Olive Oil
1 Cup Chopped Bean Sprouts
1 Cup Chopped Celery
1 Can Cream of Mushroom Soup
1 ½ Cups Uncooked Rice (not minute)
¼ Cup Soy Sauce
½ teaspoon Pepper
1 Can Dry Chinese Noodles

Brown the meat in the oil until it is crumbly, then add the sprouts, celery, soup, and water. Stir in the uncooked rice, soy sauce, and pepper. Turn into a 9x11 baking dish. Cover with foil and bake in a 350° oven for 30 minutes. Uncover and bake another 30 minutes. Cover with the Chinese noodles and bake another 15 minutes.

Crab Quiche

1 Tablespoon Butter
1 Cup Shredded Crab Meat
1 Tablespoon Flour
1 ½ Cups Coarsely Shredded Swiss Cheese, Divided
2 Tablespoons Green Onions (if you can tolerate
them, I don't use them)
9 Inch Pie Shell, Partially Baked
        (Can also use shredded potatoes, pressed like a
crust and partially baked)
3 Eggs
1 cup Light Cream, Half and Half, or Milk
        (I use non-fat organic milk)
½ teaspoon salt
Dash of White Pepper or Hot-Pepper Sauce
Dash of Nutmeg (if you can tolerate it)

Sauté the green onions (if using) in the butter, add
crab meat and flour. Set aside. Sprinkle half the
cheese in the pie shell, then spread with the crab
mixture. Sprinkle with the remaining cheese. Whisk
the eggs, cream, salt, pepper, and nutmeg (if using)
until mixed and somewhat frothy. Pour into the pie
shell and bake in pre-heated 350° oven 30-40 minutes
until set and lightly browned. A knife inserted should
come out mostly clean.

Creamed Eggs
Good for breakfast or for dinner.

6 Eggs, boiled
2 Tablespoons Flour (rice flour works)
2 Tablespoons Butter
3 Cups Milk, more or less
Salt
Pepper

Chop the boiled eggs. I prefer the whites to be in strips. Make rue by melting the butter in a sauce pan then adding the flour. Add the milk. As this begins to thicken, add the chopped eggs, whites and yolks. Salt and pepper to taste. Dish should be thickened, but somewhat pourable.

Serve over baked or boiled potatoes. This can also be served over toast.

Cranberry Juice Jellies

1 Envelope Unflavored Gelatin
8 Ounces Cranberry Juice
     (Be sure it is sweetened only with acceptable sugar)

In a small saucepan sprinkle the gelatin over the juice. Let stand one minute. Stir over low heat until the gelatin is dissolved, about 3 minutes. Pour into a small dish and chill until firm. Cut into squares or shapes for finger eating.

Fish Sauce

Mayo
Mustard (be careful of ingredients)
Worcestershire Sauce

Mix the ingredients together. Adjust by adding a bit
more if needed.

Kabobs

Steak
Mushrooms
Green Peppers
Zucchini (small ones)
Cauliflower

Cut the steak into 1 inch chunks. Slice the peppers into one inch strips, then cut them in half. The zucchini can be either sliced into rounds or cut in half lengthwise and then cut into 1 inch chunks. Use the cauliflower florets and whole mushrooms.

Place the ingredients on a kabob stick, brush with olive oil, then roast over an open fire, bar-b-que, or under the broiler.

Lettuce Wraps

Lettuce (be sure it is an acceptable one)
Homemade Mayo
Turkey Pieces (or preferred meat)
Grated Cheese or Cream Cheese
Mushrooms

Spread mayo on a lettuce leaf. Place turkey pieces, cheese, and mushrooms in a row on the leaf. Then roll the leaf burrito fashion.

If you prefer your roll warm, pre-warm the meat, but take care not to overheat it.

Macaroni, Cheese, & Broccoli

3 Cups Macaroni
1 Pound Monterey Jack Cheese, Grated
1 Can Cream of Mushroom Soup
1 Cup Sour Cream
1 Cup Cooked Broccoli Pieces
Salt & Pepper to Taste

Cook the macaroni until done. Mix the soup and sour cream together. In a casserole, start layering the ingredients with a little soup mixture in the bottom, followed by macaroni, cheese, all the broccoli, soup mixture, macaroni, cheese, and top with the soup mixture. Sprinkle with salt and pepper.

Bake at 350° until cheese melts and the casserole is bubbly.

Manicotti

8 Manicotti Shells
1 Cup Small Curd Cottage cheese
4 Ounces Mozzarella Cheese
1 Egg, Slightly Beaten
1 Tablespoon Parsley, Chopped
½ teaspoon Oregano
¼ teaspoon pepper
2 Cups Amazing Spaghetti Sauce (page 175)
Parmesan Cheese

Cook manicotti in a large amount of boiling salted water for 6 minutes. Pour off hot water and add cold water, being careful not to split the shells.

Combine the cottage cheese, mozzarella, egg, parsley, and seasonings.
Pour some of the spaghetti sauce into the bottom of a long baking dish (just enough to cover).
Fill the shells with the cheese mixture using a teaspoon or a pastry bag with a large hole. Lay the stuffed shells in a single layer in the baking dish.
Pour the sauce over the manicotti. Sprinkle with parmesan cheese. Cover with foil and bake in a 350° oven for 20 minutes. Uncover and bake 10 minutes longer or until bubbly. Let stand for 10 minutes before serving.

Mayo – Basic

1 Egg
1 Cup Olive Oil
¼ teaspoon salt
2 Tablespoons White Vinegar
Dash of Pepper or Red Pepper

Add the egg, salt, vinegar, and pepper to a blender.
Blend on High, adding oil one drop at a time at first,
slowly increasing as mixture thickens. Stop the
blender and wipe the sides, blend again. Refridgerate.

For the Advanced FMer – meaning you have
experimented and know more of the ingredients you
can tolerate:

Try substituting 1 Tablespoon of Lemon Juice for 1
Tablespoon of the Vinegar.

Try adding 1 teaspoon of dry mustard or 1/8 teaspoon
of prepared mustard (be careful of the ingredients).

Try adding ¼ teaspoon of Worcestershire sauce.

Meatloaf

3 Slices Bread (or equal amount in crumbs)
¾ Cup Milk
2 Eggs
5 Soda Crackers (crumbled)
2 ½ Pound Ground Meat
      (we used 1 ½ lb. beef & 1 lb. buffalo)
1 stalk Celery, diced or chopped
1 Can Mushrooms
1 ½ teaspoon Salt
½ teaspoon Sage
½ teaspoon Dry Mustard
½ teaspoon Pepper
1½ Tablespoon Worcestershire Sauce
6 Slices Uncured Bacon
Banana Ketchup (optional)

Dry the bread to make crumbs. Mix all the ingredients together except the Banana Ketchup. Divide into two loaf pans (or scoop into cupcake pan for individual servings). Bake at 350 for an hour (less for cupcake pan).

Omelet – Basic

2 Eggs
2 Tablespoons Water
¼ teaspoon Salt
Dash of Pepper or Tabasco
½ Tablespoon Butter

Topping Possibilities:
Cheese
Uncured Bacon
Spinach
Bean Sprouts
Zucchini
Broccoli
Use your imagination!

Heat the butter in an 8 or 10 in non-stick skillet.

Place first four ingredients in a bowl and whisk until it begins to be frothy.

Pour the egg mixture into the medium-hot skillet. With the pancake turner keep pushing the sides of the egg toward the center until the runny egg stops flowing out to the edge. Turn down to medium-low. Add the cheese (if using) on the whole egg, followed by any other topping on one side of the egg only. When the egg top is slightly moist, fold the omelet in half. Flip or slide onto a plate. The omelet is best if allow to sit for a minute or two before serving.

Peanut Butter Logs

1 Tablespoon Cane Sugar
2 Tablespoons Peanut Butter
2-3 Tablespoons Nonfat Dry Milk
Chopped Nuts (optional)

Blend the sugar and peanut butter in a bowl with a wooden spoon. Add the dry milk. Make a dry still paste. Shape the paste into balls or roll into one long log to cut into one inch bite size logs. Roll in nuts, if using. Wrap. Chill in the refrigerator.

Pork Noodle Stir-Fry

9 Ounces thin Chinese-style egg noodles
4 Tablespoons Olive Oil
1 ½ Pound Pork, cut into julienne strips
1 Cup Bean Sprouts
¼ Cup Shredded Fresh Basil
3 Tablespoons Pine Nuts, toasted
        Careful, they burn easily
2 Tablespoons Balsamic Vinegar
Sea Salt to Taste
Ground Pepper to Taste

Cook the noodles in a large saucepan of boiling water until done. Drain, the toss with 2 tablespoons of olive oil.

Coat the hot wok with 2 tablespoons of olive oil. Add the Pork, cooking for 2-3 minutes. Add the bean sprouts, then stir-fry for a minute.

Add basil, pine nuts, and balsamic vinegar. Mix well, then add the noodles, salt, and pepper and toss.

Potato Pancakes

3 Cups Mashed Potatoes
2 Well Beaten Eggs
1 ½ Tablespoons Flour
1/8 teaspoon baking powder
1 teaspoon salt
¼ Cup Green Onions (if you tolerate)

Mix together all ingredients. Spoon onto hot skillet as you would pancake batter. Flip when brown on bottom.

Potato Salad

6 Medium Potatoes
½ Cup Chopped Bean Sprouts (optional)
1 teaspoon Salt
1/8 teaspoon Pepper
¼ Cup Italian Salad Dressing, or Oil and Balsamic
Vinegar
½ Cup Mayonnaise
½ Cup Chopped Celery
3-4 Hard Boiled Eggs-Chopped

Mix the first five ingredients together and let set the
refrigerator overnight. Add the remaining ingredients
and mix. This is best is allowed to refrigerate at this
point for at least 4, preferably 8 hours.

Salmon & Vegetables at the Ranch

2 Salmon Fillets
¼ teaspoon lemon
¼ Cup Ranch Dressing (be careful)
3 Cups Vegetables
      Broccoli, Cauliflower, and Sugar Snap Peas
all work well
½ teaspoon ground basil
Salt to Taste
Pepper to Taste

Rub the lemon juice on the bottom of an oven-safe dish. Add the salmon. Spread the ranch dressing over the fillets. Sprinkle with half the spices. Top with the chopped vegetables. Sprinkle with other half of the spices. Cover with a lid or foil.

Bake 15-18 minutes or until salmon flakes easily with a fork.

Scalloped Potatoes

6 Medium Potatoes
Salt & Pepper to Taste
2 Tablespoons Flour
4 Tablespoons Butter
Milk
Add cheese for au'graten

Peel the raw potatoes and cut into thin slices. Place a
layer of potatoes in the baking dish 1 inch deep.
Season with salt and pepper, sprinkle a portion of the
flour over each layer, add a part of the butter in bits.
Repeat and continue until required amount is used.
Best not to have more than two or three layers. Add
milk until it can be seen between the slices of
potatoes. Cover and bake at 350° - 400°until the
potatoes are tender when pierced with a fork, 1-1 ½
hours. Remove the cover during the last 15 minutes.

Shrimp Salad

2 Cups Uncooked Shell Macaroni
3 Boiled Eggs, Diced
½ Cup Diced Celery
¼ Cup Chopped Bean Sprouts (optional)
½ to 1 Cup Cocktail Shrimp
¼ to ½ Cup Tiny Broccoli Floret Pieces
        (or whatever green veggie you would like to
use, it originally uses peas)
Salt to Taste
Pepper to Taste

Cook the macaroni, then drain and rinse well with
cold water. Mix all the ingredients well. Refrigerate
for 4-8 hours before serving.

Spread

1 Small Can Chopped Green Chilies
½ Cup Mayo
½ Cup Cream Cheese
½ Cup Grated Monterey Jack Cheese

Mix ingredients well. Spread on bread or crackers and broil until lightly browned on top.

This works well for pizza sauce if you leave out the cheese..

Stuffed Potatoes

Baked Potatoes

Your choices of:
>Butter
>Uncured Bacon
>Cheese
>Cream Cheese
>Broccoli
>Zucchini
>Cauliflower
>Sour Cream

Salt & Pepper to Taste

Cut the baked potato length-wise and fill with your favorite toppings.

Tater Tot Casserole

1 Large Package Tater Tots
        (read ingredients, many have unwanted items)
1-2 Cups Chopped, Cooked Chicken or Turkey
1 Cup Chopped Broccoli, Fresh or Frozen
        (or Edimame, Cauliflower, etc.)
½ to 1 Cup Grated Cheese (optional)
½ Cup Stock or Bouillon
1 Can Cream of Mushroom Soup
½ Cup Sour Cream

Place the tater tots in a 9x13 baking dish, top with the chicken, and follow this with the broccoli and cheese, if using. Mix the stock, soup, and sour cream thoroughly. Spread this mixture evenly over the tater tot mixture.

Bake in a 350° oven for one hour.

Wild Turkey Surprise

3 Cups Cooked White Rice
1 Cup Celery, Sliced
1 Can Cream of Mushroom Soup, Diluted with ½ Cup Water
½ teaspoon Salt
¼ teaspoon Pepper
2-2 ½ Cups Chopped Chicken or Turkey
1 Cup Cheese, Grated
¼ Cup Dry White Wine
½ Cup Sour Cream

In a very large skillet, sauté the celery in butter until it is tender. Add the soup, water, sour cream, wine, salt, and pepper. Stir well and let heat for a bit, but do not let it boil. Add the chicken, heat, but do not boil. Stir the rice into this mixture. Pour the mixture into a large shallow baking dish. Sprinkle with the cheese.

Bake, uncovered, for 20 minutes at 350°.

Sources

Works Cited:

[1.] Barrett, Jacqueline S. & Gibson (sic?), Peter R. "Clinical Ramifications of Malabsorption   of Fructose and Other Short Chain Carbohydrates" Practical Gastroenterology,   August 2007. January 2008
        http://www.healthsystem.virginia.edu/internet/ digestive-health/nutrition/BarrettArticle.pdf

[2]. Corn Refiners Association "Nutritive Sweeteners from Corn" 2006, February 2008
http://www.corn.org/NSFC2006.pdf

[3]. Gotze, H. & Mahdi A., Comment in Monatsschr Kinderheilkd (German, translated),   April 1993, February 2008
        http://www.ncbi.nlm.nih.gov/pubmed/1470188 ?dopt=A

[4]. Kosmix Right Health, accessed February 2008
        http://www.righthealth.com/Health/High__fru ctose__corn__syrup/-od-
definition_wiki_High__fructose__corn__syrup-s

[5]. Ledochowski, Maximilian, Überall, Florian, Propst, Theresia, & Fuchs, Dietmar   "Fructose Malabsorption Is Associated with Lower Plasma Folic

Acid   Concentrations in Middle-Aged Subjects"
Clinical Chemistry 1999, February   2008
http://www.clinchem.org/cgi/content/full/45/11/2013

[6]. Natoli, Sharon, "Fructose Malabsorption" Medical
Observer, April 2006. February 2008
        <http://www.medicalobserver.com.au/displaya
rticle/index.asp?articleID=6260&templateID=108&se
ctionID=0&sectionName=

[7]. University of Virginia, Digestive Health Center
"Low Fructose Diet" accessed February   2008
<http://www.healthsystem.virginia.edu/internet/digest
ive-   health/nutrition/low-fructose-diet.pdf
[8]. Nutritional Research Center.Org, "Health Tip #3",
http://nutritionresearchcenter.org/healthnews/health-
tip-3-nix-high-fructose-corn-syrup/

[9]. Christian Antonioli, *PhD candidate in psychiatry*[1],
Michael A Reveley, *professor of psychiatry*[1 (june 2005)]

[10]. Niedzielin K, Kordecki H, Birkenfeld B (2001).
"A controlled, double-blind, randomized study on the
efficacy of Lactobacillus plantarum 299V in patients
with irritable bowel syndrome". *Eur J Gastroenterol
Hepatol* **13** (10): 1143–7. doi:10.1097/00042737-
200110000-00004. PMID 11711768.
http://meta.wkhealth.com/pt/pt-core/template-
journal/lwwgateway/media/landingpage.htm?issn=09
54-691X&volume=13&issue=10&spage=1143.

[11.] Boston University, HFI Laboratory
http://www.bu.edu/aldolase/HFI/treatment/sugar_table.htm

[12.] Prevention Magazine, March 2009, page 48

[13.] http://www.pulsus.com/cddw2007/abs/229
Fructose Malabsorption May Be Gender
Dependent and Fails to Show Compensation by
Colonic Adaptation, A Szilagyi, P Malolepszy, S
Yesovitch, C Vinokuroff, U Nathwani, A Cohen,
X Xue
Division of Gastroenterology, Department of
Medicine, Department of Dietetics and
Department of Emergency Medicine, Sir Mortimer
B Davis Jewish General Hospital, McGill
University, Montreal, Quebec

Other sources:

http://www.psychologyinfo.com/depression/

http://www.nimh.nih.gov/publicat/depression.cfm

http://www.dbsalliance.org/WPsearchable.pdf

http://www.mixednuts.net/depression-famous2.html

http://www.efmoody.com/longterm/depression.html

http://weblinks1.epnet.com GETTING DOWN TO
DEPRESSION , By: Salmans, Sandra, Depression:
Questions You Have...Answers You Need, 1997

FDA Consumer, May-June 2006

Harvard School of Public Health
http://www.hsph.harvard.edu/nutritionsource
and
www.thenutritionsource.org

Journal of Food Science
http://www3.interscience.wiley.com/journal/1188324
76/abstract

The World's Healthiest Foods website
http://whfoods.org/genpage.php?tname=nutrient&dbid
=103#foodsources

http://www.raisin-hell.com/2008/11/fructans-

inulin.html

http://www.sciencedaily.com/releases/2009/04/09042
0182151.htm

http://news.health.ufl.edu/news/story.aspx?ID=4992

Index

Made in the USA
Charleston, SC
02 April 2013